The
Woman's
Herbal
Apothecary

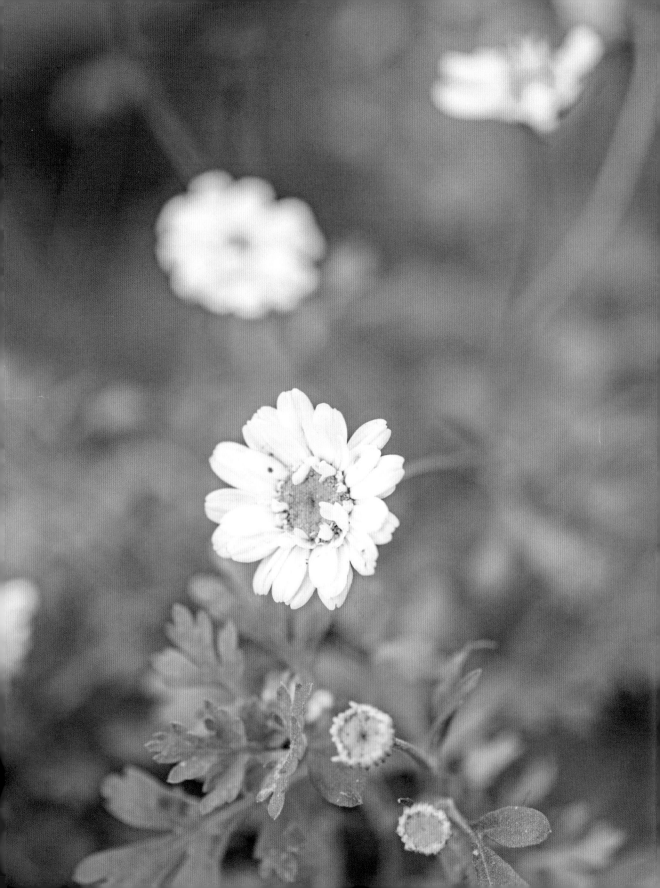

The Woman's Herbal Apothecary

200 Natural Remedies for Healing, Hormone Balance,
Beauty and Longevity, and Creating Calm

JJ PURSELL

FAIR WINDS

Quarto.com

© 2018 Quarto Publishing Group USA Inc.
Text © 2018 JJ Pursell
Photography © 2018 Shawn Linehan

First Published in 2018 by Fair Winds Press, an imprint of The Quarto Group,
100 Cummings Center, Suite 265-D, Beverly, MA 01915, USA.
T (978) 282-9590 F (978) 283-2742

Fair Winds Press titles are also available at discount for retail, wholesale, promotional, and bulk purchase. For details, contact the Special Sales Manager by email at specialsales@quarto.com or by mail at The Quarto Group, Attn: Special Sales Manager, 100 Cummings Center, Suite 265-D, Beverly, MA 01915, USA.

25   7

ISBN: 978-1-59233-820-7

Digital edition published in 2018
eISBN: 978-1-63159-465-6

Library of Congress Cataloging-in-Publication Data

Pursell, J. J., 1973- author.
The woman's herbal apothecary : 100 natural remedies for healing,
   hormone balance, beauty and longevity, and creating calm / JJ Pursell.
ISBN 9781592338207 (paperback)
1. Herbs--Therapeutic use. 2. Women--Health and hygiene.
RM666.H33 P874 2018
615.3/21--dc23
2018012265

Cover Design: Kate Barraclough
Interior Design and page layout: Allison Meierding
Photography: Shawn Linehan
Illustration: Abby Diamond | @Finchfight

Printed in China

The information in this book is for educational purposes only. It is not intended to replace the advice of a physician or medical practitioner. Please see your health-care provider before beginning any new health program.

This book is dedicated to my children, Cordelia and Tommy.

May the plants always whisper their secrets to you and

may you grow up to be healthy and wise in the ways

of independence and equality.

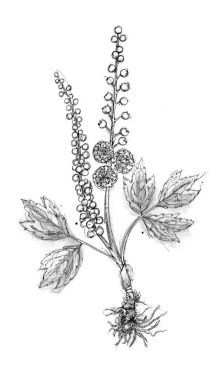

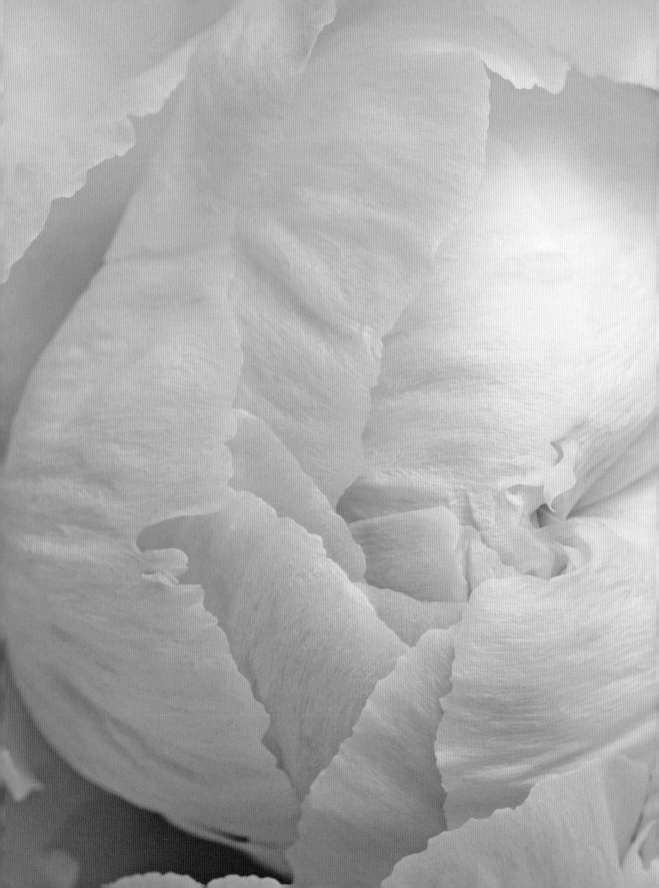

Contents

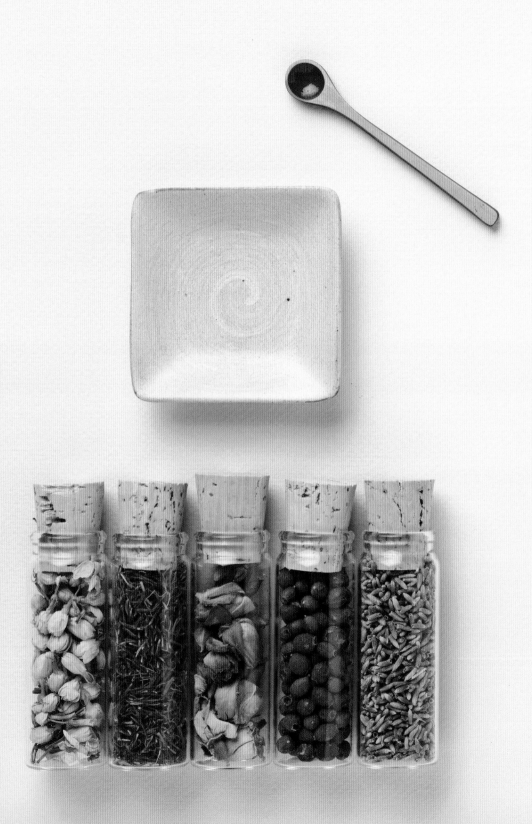

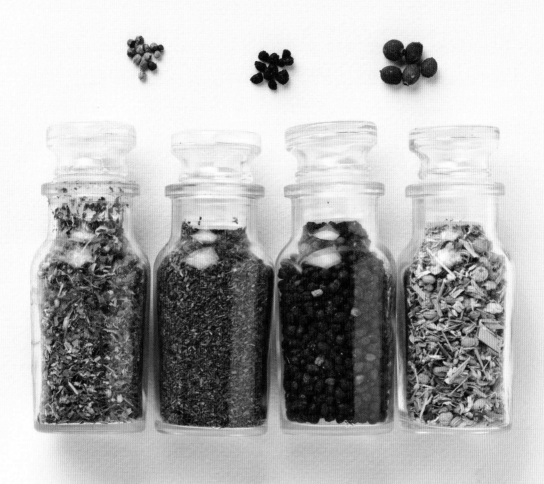

Introduction

LEARNING ABOUT HERBS felt to me like remembering something from long ago. Everything I read made sense both logically and intuitively. Although I grew up loving science, it was always something I had to work hard to fully comprehend. This was different. The information flowed in and miraculously stayed. Not only that, I could access it whenever I needed it. It was a love affair of sorts—and one I've held in wonder. I hesitate to use the word *magic*, but to me that is what herbal medicine manifests. Once I opened my herb shop and began to teach about herbs, I noticed the same thing was happening with my students. I call it *the herbal awakening*. I start each new herb class by asking students what brought them to it. Most want to help themselves and others, and using herbs just makes sense to them.

If you go to any herb conference, women will most likely surround you. Many men have also embraced herbal studies of course, but women seem to have a strong calling to it. Even though women have historically been restricted from training at the schools of medicines, they have always been the lifeblood of the home, farm, and community. Knowing that yarrow flower tea could be used to break a fever, for example, or that wormwood would dispel worms from the body was imperative to survival. In fact, herbs were so important in many circles that they were viewed as sacred, and only an indoctrinated priestess could gather them. When you're out in the woods, away from it all, it is easy to visualize that beautiful blend of gathering healing plants and ritual, and that era doesn't seem far away.

There are countless books on the history and usage of herbs in various cultures. Much of the information they contain is still relevant today or can be easily modernized. It has led to the creation of pharmacognosy, the branch of knowledge concerned with medicinal drugs obtained from plants or other natural resources. Today, we can all give thanks to healing plants and the scientists that study them. Many of our modern life-saving medications originated from them. The key to consider here, though, is that herbs, in their natural state, still work. Although science has expanded by leaps and bounds, discarding the use of herbs in their whole form is shortsighted. Having a well-rounded education in both modern and traditional medicine creates a treasure trove of options.

It can be difficult to stand up for what we believe in, whether it is how we choose to care for ourselves or against any type of injustice. Finding communities to support us can be hard. Our society's view of women, for example, needs to be reshaped.

Addressing discrimination effectively has proven challenging and is often met with judgment. But strengthening and unifying our female communities through self-acceptance is one way to shift the current paradigm. That is what this book is all about: teaching you about your body, showing you how to care for it naturally, and encouraging you to know yourself inside and out. When we do this, our power increases. Your decisions are driven by who you really are, not by what society expects you to be or do. Your self-worth is a measurement you create while striving to be the best you can be without allowing others to weigh in. When we view ourselves as worthy, we afford others the same respect. When we view ourselves as worthy, great things can happen, and we can allow ourselves to be seen and shared with the world.

The Woman's Herbal Apothecary teaches the foundations of herbal medicine and women's health. The words *women* and *woman* are not intended to limit those lessons to those who have an anatomical uterus. I use these words to impart feminine energy, power, and healing to anyone who wishes them. If you are looking for herbal guidance and have an anatomical uterus, but you don't relate to the word *woman*, you can still use this information to care for your physical body. I honor my womanhood and balanced masculinity and femininity, so this book is written from that perspective, but I do not intend to exclude anyone from the healing wisdom of herbs with the language I use.

This book will guide you through the years of your life, offering insights and self-care all along the way. I've also included pearls of health so that you can fully understand how the female physical body works and functions. The more we know, the more empowered we are and the less room there is for fear, shock, or bewilderment when our body starts to act in a new way. It is my hope that the information contained within these pages will empower you in a multitude of ways. Perhaps it will unlock the passions of herbal medicine or provide you with the support you need to honor all of your glorious body. At the very least, it should give you plenty of context to know your body better and to support it from day to day.

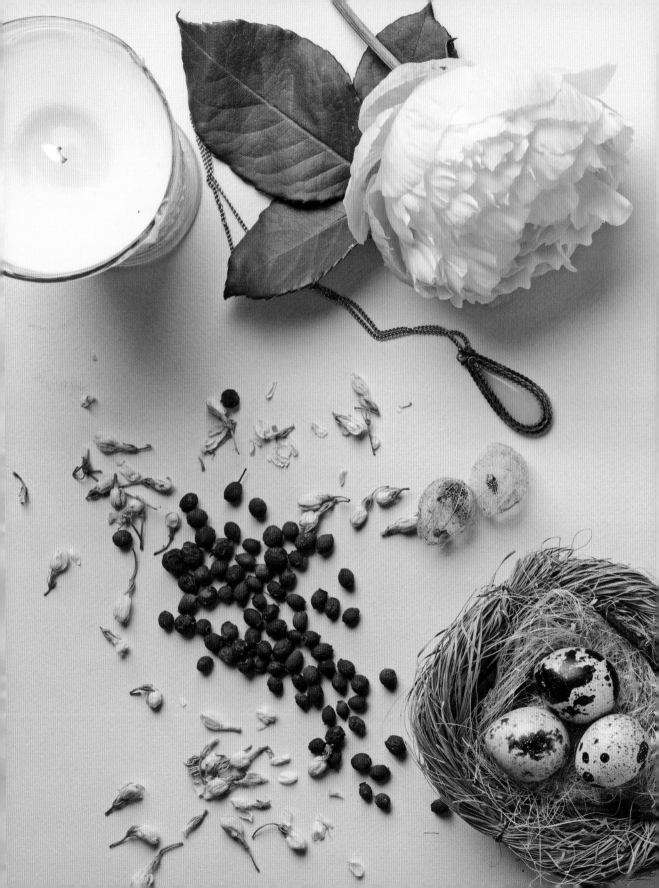

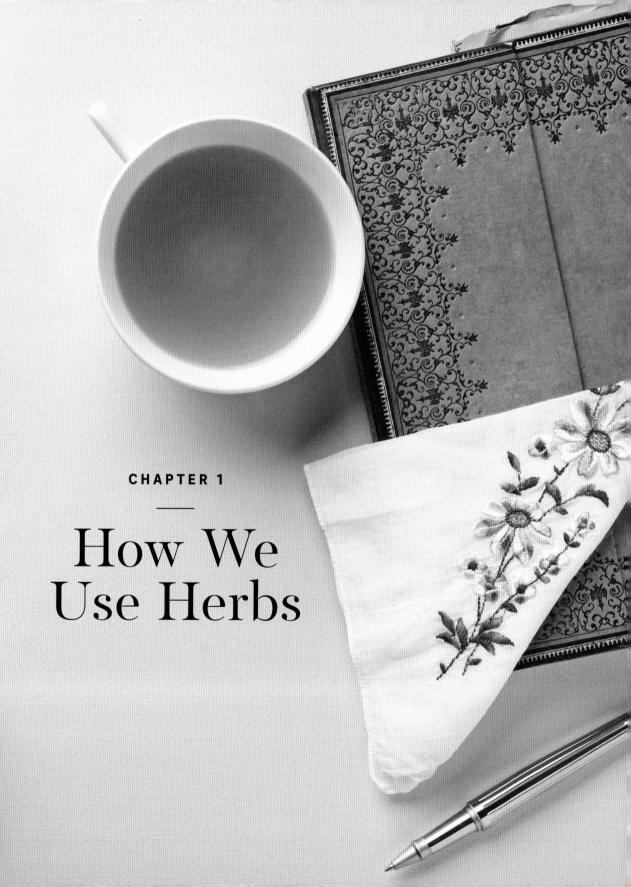

CHAPTER 1

How We
Use Herbs

WELCOME TO THE WORLD OF HERBS! These pages contain endless opportunities for you to learn about the healing arts of herbal medicine. When we learn how to use herbs in our daily lives, we are creating a relationship and a higher level of confidence with our body. Make this book your go-to for how to support and care for a woman's body. I encourage you to feel safe enough to try the recipes. Even if you haven't used herbs before, I'm going to give you the guidance you need to jump in.

I've been using and practicing herbal medicine for more than twenty-five years. I've worked on herb farms, in herb shops, and in practice as a naturopath/ acupuncturist/herbalist. But all that began one winter day after I had just moved to the Pacific Northwest. I was a young, interested herbalist simply standing in my kitchen, looking at vitex berries. I'd read they were supposed to help regulate the menstrual cycle, something I'd been struggling with. But now what? I looked at the little plastic bag that had 1 ounce (28 g) of berries in it and decided to dump them into a bowl. I smelled them and even tasted one, and then I decided to make a tea per the instructions I had received from my local herb shop. Mind you, at the time I was used to tea bag tea that came perfectly blended to please my palate. What I quickly learned from drinking this vitex tea is that there was a whole range of taste that I'd never known. And that was it—my first experience with herbs. Your first experience may be that simple, or it may be more like the time I decided to brew hops for a bedtime tea and steeped it for fifteen minutes. It was far too bitter to drink! But it is still a funny experience to think about. You're not always going to get it right the first time when you are learning something new. But isn't that the point? It's the act of trying that's so important. You can do this, just as I did many, many years ago.

This book is meant to be a resource, a platform upon which to learn to use herbs in a safe and respectful way. It is not meant to cure disease or replace the relationship you have with your health care provider. I'm striving to educate and encourage women to have a deeper relationship with themselves using self-care, herbal medicine, and bodily knowledge. We live in a modern medical era, and most of us have the privilege of living in a developed country with access to health care. Please use it when needed. And for the in-between times, enjoy the process of learning how to better care for yourself on a day-to-day basis.

First, we'll go through how to use herbs for healing. What is a tincture? A poultice? Knowing the different application types gives you a foundation upon which to build.

Then we will discuss the language of herbal medicine. Is an herb a sedative or a stimulant? Does is calm the digestive system? That is a *carminative*. Knowing these definitions gives you a clear idea of what each herb may or may not do in the body. The table on page 25 includes the original apothecary terms used during the times of Nicholas Culpepper, the famous herbalist of the 1600s, which are still used today. If you have a background or interest in science, the "Herbal Bio Constituents" section will peak your curiosity; it is a brief introduction to the scientific nature of plant components extracted into their individual parts. It is these individual parts that have been used repeatedly in pharmacology to make modern medications. Having a general idea of all the above gives you a solid background in how plants are studied and most often used. But it is in the herbal *materia medica* where you will begin to acquaint yourself with the plants. A materia medica is a medical list of healing agents. For our purposes, the materia medica is a list of herbs that are specific to women's health. It was created to give you a closer glimpse at the herbs that are most often referenced throughout the rest of the book.

POSITIVE FEMININE PRACTICES

Before we get into the education portion of this chapter, I'd like to share with you a group of modalities that I refer to as Positive Feminine Practices. This is a group of practices I've collected over the years that I've found to be beneficial for balancing women's health, emotions, and energy. They are things I've personally practiced and have offered to others. Herbal medicine is a wonderful tool in our health and healing toolbox, but having an overflowing toolbox gives us an abundance of options to choose from and try.

As we move through life, it gets busy and full, and we often get distracted. I was recently reminded of a truth I often forget. We busy ourselves to keep from having to see, feel, and be who we really are. Finding time to return to daily care, let alone to connect to ourselves and others, can be challenging. Here is my hope for you: Remember your strengths daily. Give thanks for all that you have, even when it doesn't feel like much. Drench yourself in a feeling of love and radiance for one minute every evening. Get a photo of yourself and collage all around it with healing, healthy words and pictures of things you love. Look at it daily. Make this a meditation. You are beautiful, and it's time you honor that.

I've used several different techniques to help me reconnect over the years. As someone who tends to veer off path when I get overworked, overstressed, or distracted by someone else's needs, I need gentle practice to reclaim myself and my balance. When I was struggling with my irregular menses cycles, one of the first techniques I used was exercise. (You can read the full story in chapter 3.) I turned to basic forms of yoga in an attempt to create Zen and flexibility—literally and figuratively—in my chaotic life. I didn't care that I was in sweatpants while everyone else looked like a yoga model; it felt *good*. In the stretching and pulling of different body parts, I felt as though my body began to breathe again. Through conversations in class I was encouraged to find the book *Luna Yoga* by Adelheid Ohlig. It's an incredible little book, originally published in Germany, that features yoga poses specifically for balancing hormones and the menstrual cycle. The practice allowed room for femininity as I stretched to the moon or rang my womb like a bell. The poses were strange, and at times I found myself laughing as I learned to move my hips in ways I never had before—all in the name of bringing vital energy and circulation to the abdomen and pelvic region. I loved it! It also combined the massage of certain acupuncture points in conjunction with the poses. Because I was embarking on my study of Chinese medicine, I was even more motivated to carve time out of my schedule for a daily practice. Although I hadn't ever imagined doing it before, I now couldn't imagine living without it.

Another yoga form I really took to was kundalini. I went to my first class on a whim and left feeling like I could breathe one hundred pounds more air per minute. Kundalini involves movement, breathing techniques, meditation, and the chanting of mantras. Chanting of mantras? Who had I become? But yes; after a few short weeks I was belting them out and feeling phenomenal. Typically, each class would focus on one bodily system, for example the immune system or the digestive system, while doing repetitive exercises for several minutes at a time. This repetitive motion often created a meditation without even trying. Another benefit of kundalini? You rest between each exercise! You actually lie down and just *be* for a few minutes. Glorious!

Whether it's a quiet practice such as yoga or a vibrant burst of running, keep in mind that exercise is important for women. I know not everyone likes to "exercise," but I find it hard to believe that there is someone who doesn't feel better from even the simplest of daily movements. Walking your dog or taking a walk with a friend after dinner can have powerful effects. I used to walk my dog daily when I lived in the city.

I walked that route every day. It allowed me time to reflect on the seasons and my life. And sometimes I walked the entire way on autopilot, obviously processing and clearing out thoughts that needed to be free. Find your movement must-have and commit to it regularly; it truly is one of the best ways to tap into yourself.

If you haven't familiarized yourself with Vikki Noble, I would highly suggest it. She singlehandedly changed my life through the introduction of Shakti, in her book *Shakti Woman*. I often think about the opening of that book now, more than twenty years later. In it she describes the moment she told her young children that going forward she would no longer be available in the morning hours because she was beginning a meditation practice. They would be responsible for getting themselves prepared for school. What a brave and defining moment of self-reclaiming. My mornings currently look like someone has just shot the race gun off and I'm already behind. Although I can't manifest two hours of quiet upon rising, remembering the lessons of the Shakti woman have helped me return to balance over and over throughout the years.

Another tradition I consider myself fortunate to have experienced and trained in is the tradition of Mayan abdominal massage (see chapter 3). Rosita Arvigo, founder of the Arvigo Institute, is an American woman who has led seminars in this healing technique for more than thirty years. I'll let you discover Rosita's story on your own, but her practice is founded on the physical centering of the uterus in a woman's body. It is said that if a woman's uterus is midline and center, then she herself is acting from a centered place. The techniques are helpful for both physical and emotional ailments centered on the female reproductive system.

Journaling is another way to pull swirls of emotion from the inside to the outside. You don't need any skill or art to journal; you must only do it. I often find that having no censor is the best way for me to access myself. I'll begin by free-writing, which manifests most often as a stream of consciousness, simply writing down whatever comes out. Through this process, I can move my thinking brain off the stage and let my subconscious take over. When I get done, it's as though I've just had a therapy session; I'm often surprised at what has been bubbling below the surface. I've even taken to blogging anonymously at times for emotional release, particularly during heavy computer project times. If something comes up, I can quickly open a browser tab and spit out whatever is gnawing at me. This makes it easier to move on because I've acknowledged it, no matter how pretty or ugly it may be. The simple act of allowing yourself the freedom to feel whatever is going on in your life allows for forgiveness, growth, and self-acceptance.

I love a good collage session and am repeatedly surprised at what manifests from one. Collaging or vision boarding is a way to help you see what is holding you back, what you want out of life, what you hope to achieve—really anything you set your intention to be. Find a piece of paper or poster board and collect lots of magazines from friends and family. Choose a quiet time and make a cup of tea. Sit for a few moments and decide what you want out of the experience. As you move through it, it may change, and that is okay. The exercise itself helps clear the cobwebs of doubt, insecurity, or lack of confidence in what you deserve and can achieve. To begin, cut out pictures and words of what you are focused on. This is a fun activity with kids too, as it gives them a new way to express themselves before their emotional and verbal communication skills have been refined. You can also draw on the board. Sometimes, I'll create a dream board with the intention of trying to achieve certain things in my life, and as time goes by, I realize what is on my board isn't quite right. That's when I find another picture or word and add it to the board. Use collaging to get out of your head—to discover what is holding you back and where you are meant to go.

Now is the time to begin to learn about the magic of herbal medicine and to connect what you learn to who you really are. The two go hand in hand. Together, they encourage self-confidence and the knowledge that you are worth caring for.

HOW DO WE USE HERBAL MEDICINE?

What does it mean to be an herbalist? There is no right answer to this question. You get to decide for yourself what it means. For me, it has meant different things at different times. When I first started learning about herbs, it was a title I never felt good enough for. The term *herbalist* was reserved for those in the field who had been using and teaching herbs for years. But after some time passed and my friends all kept calling me an herbalist, I realized I *was* an herbalist. I was using herbs to help my body and mind feel good daily. I could identify herbs in the wild, and I knew how to blend a tea and make a tincture. I'm not sure why I wouldn't allow myself to be called an herbalist before that. I think our society puts emphasis on certain labels, and I had followed suit, deciding the term *herbalist* designated only those with a mastery in the field. The truth is, anyone is an herbalist if he or she is studying and using plants as medicine. Claim the title. It's your right.

Many people I speak with want to know how to work with people as an herbalist. At my shop, Fettle Botanic Supply & Counsel, we often counsel customers with our herbal references. By utilizing our textbooks and herbal references, we work in tandem with our customers to identify the problem and curate an herbal solution, if one is available. Seeing clients as an herbalist is a responsibility not to be taken lightly.

Many people consider herbs benign and harmless, but education and experience are necessary when working with medicinal plants. That said, if your heart and mind are ready to offer such services, I encourage you to do so. Working with clients in a counseling environment is a great way to offer services to others in regard to their health. I often find that those who seek out herbal treatments enjoy the opportunity to work with a practitioner to create the right blends. For more, check out Margi Flint's incredible book *The Practicing Herbalist*, which focuses on how to set up and run an herbal clinic. There are also many online and at-home natural health courses available, but not all of them are what I'd consider a high enough caliber to train you to work with clients. There are, however, many courses that go above and beyond in their trainings, and I've listed some later in the book. Should you find your love of herbs bleeding into your passion for helping others heal, offer your gifts to the world. My advice: Listen intently to your clients and never stop your learning path.

In this book, I'll be focusing on how to use herbs to be the best you can be. This means feeling your best on the inside, which leads to looking your best on the outside. In herbal medicine, we use different application types when using herbs for our body or soul. The application type you choose depends on what you are aiming to accomplish. A topical application is often used for skin, but there are times when an internal treatment such as a tea or tincture is necessary to correct internal imbalance so that the skin can glow. Other times, using two different application types at the same time can result in an efficient, quick result. One example would be when you are experiencing stress: You can combine a tincture for incredibly stressful moments with a daily tea that works on the underlying foundations of stress reduction and nourishment of the stress centers.

Let's review the different herbal application types to better understand how herbs are used. Although this is not the end-all list of how you can use herbs, these are the most common ways used in today's households. That said, I know I'm not alone in my love of reading the classic texts of herbalism and learning different and unique ways to experience herbs.

PREPARATION TYPES

- Tea
- Tincture
- Poultice
- Fomentation
- Capsules

- Sitz bath
- Topical wash
- Herbal oil
- Salve

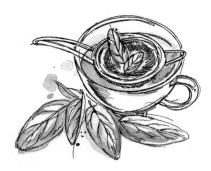

How Long Will It Take?

A tonic recipe—in tea, tincture, or capsule form—is typically taken 6 to 12 weeks. Acute recipes, such as for menstrual cramps, are taken as needed. It is best to give a new recipe a minimum of 2 to 3 weeks to see effectiveness. Hormone recipes may need 6 to 12 weeks.

If you notice side effects soon after beginning a new recipe, stop and reexamine. Is your dosage too high and you perhaps need to start at a lower dose?

If you have diagnosed health conditions, please consult with your health provider before beginning new herbal treatments.

Tea

Tea may be the oldest and most traditional form of herbal use. There is nothing simpler than placing herbs in a cup and pouring hot water over them. These days, the herbs are even conveniently packaged in neat little tea bags. I won't lie; I have a few herbal teas in tea bags that I just can't live without, but if I had to choose either bagged or bulk tea, I would most assuredly go with bulk. After all, the bulk has nothing that separates me from my medicine. I can see the herbs, watch them float around and sink to the bottom.

I can control how much I want to use, and—my favorite part—there is no packaging waste.

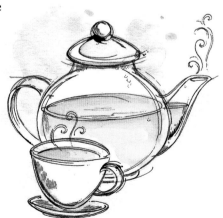

Bulk teas are often fresher, better smelling, and much more cost-efficient. There is no reason to be afraid of bulk tea and a tea ball. In fact, my guess is that it won't take long for you to fall in love with the ritual of using both.

Tincture

Tinctures are herbs that have steeped in what is called a *menstruum*. A menstruum is a liquid base that works as a solvent to break apart the herb's cell walls and extract the medicinal components of the plant. Basically, you are turning something solid into a liquid through the process of extraction. The most commonly used menstruum is a mixture of alcohol and water. Many of the medicinal components of herbs are soluble in alcohol; it's an incredible preservative, and it diffuses directly into our bloodstream for quick effect. You can also use other things, such as apple cider vinegar or vegetable glycerin (or a little of both combined for fun), but not all plants can successfully extract in either of these. If you are really excited about solubility and the biochemistry of tinctures, I suggest studying the "Herbal Bio Constituents" section on page 33 to learn what is soluble in what.

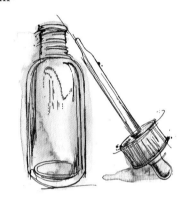

Poultice

Poultices are wonderful topical applications with strong effects. I refer to them as herb cakes. They are moistened herbs formed and patted down over the area where needed. Think of them as healing herbal Band-Aids. Most commonly you'll place whole or powdered herbs in a bowl and add just enough hot water to make them really stick together. Then you'll apply it topically where needed. Utilizing medical gauze or a bandana to hold the poultice in place is helpful. Poultices are good for stings, bites, wounds, broken bones, infection, boils, in-grown issues, acne, and anything that needs to be drawn from the skin.

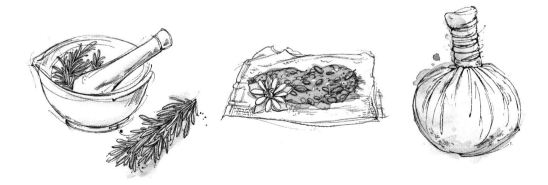

Fomentation

Fomentation is another topical application utilizing a steep infusion of herbs, typically much steeper than you would drink. After straining, you soak a cloth in the infusion and apply it to the area where needed. Fomentations are great when you need to wrap a body part or treat a large area.

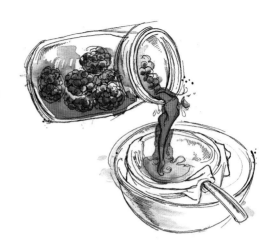

Capsules

Herbal capsules dominate the market, but they are extremely easy and much more cost-efficient to make at home. They are great for travel and for the beginning herbalist who isn't yet comfortable with the other application forms. They have no taste, which is a big plus when you are working with powerfully flavored herbs. They are perhaps not the ideal choice if your digestion system is compromised, because you want to break down the capsule and assimilate the herbs through the digestive processes. If you don't have a healthy digestive system, you won't be able to break down the capsule and it will simply be flushed out as waste.

Sitz Bath

A sitz bath is an old treatment in which you submerge your bottom and pelvis region to heal ailments in the area. The basin is filled with a warm herbal infusion that varies depending on what is being treated. I recommend using a footbath or dishwashing basin, but there are also basins that fit into the seat of the toilet. They're wonderful for postpartum healing, hemorrhoids, pelvic congestion, vaginal infection, lower back pain, and more.

Topical Wash

Topical washes are similar to fomentations, but instead of soaking a cloth and applying it to the area, you actually soak the body part in the infusion. I often use this application with my patients for pink eye (a.k.a. conjunctivitis) and eczema. For the former, I make a steep infusion and then douse the eyes several times a day with it. For the latter, I recommend infusing the herbs, straining them, and then soaking the affected area, often the hands or feet. The direct contact allows the herbs to penetrate in a unique way.

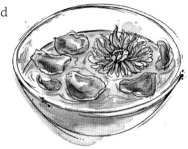

Herbal Oil

An herbal oil is made when herbs are "baked" in a base oil. The base oil is most often olive oil, but you can also use sweet almond, apricot, jojoba, avocado, grapeseed, or

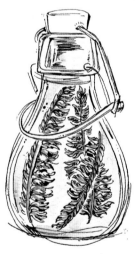

hemp oil. You can use fresh or dried plant material, and you can use the sun or the oven as your heat source. The heat works to extract the oil-soluble healing components of the herbs to create a healing herbal oil. Herbal oils are often used to make other herbal products such as salves, lotions, or creams, but they can be used just as well on their own. Remember, herbal oils and essential oils are not the same thing. Essential oils are the pure volatile oil extracted from plants, often through distillation.

Salve

An herbal healing salve is a topical treatment with a consistency similar to that of a balm or an ointment. It is often used to soothe the skin after a burn, bite, sting, abrasion, or other surface problem. Typically, it is made by adding beeswax to an herbal oil until the mixture reaches the desired consistency. I have salves all over my house—one in the kitchen for burns, one in the bathroom for boo-boos, one in the garden for nicks and cuts, and on and on.

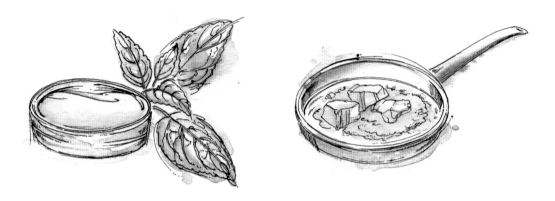

UNDERSTANDING HERBAL LANGUAGE

It's important to learn the verbiage or language associated with any new subject you take up. Without it, your ability to relate to and define the material becomes difficult. Here are two terms to know when it comes to herbal medicine: What the herbs do is defined by their *herbal action*. Herbal actions (see page 25) categorize herbs into groupings. *Herbal bio constituents* (see page 33) are how herbs are classified by scientific action in the body.

Knowing herbs by their Latin names is also extremely valuable. I can't tell you how many times someone has come into my shop requesting an herb by a name I've never heard of. Herbs are often named regionally, with the same herb growing one state over called something completely different. This is when the Latin name is vitally important. Another advantage to knowing Latin names is communication when you are traveling. Many years ago, I contracted a stomach bug in Budapest. I headed to the nearest herbal pharmacy and asked for *Ulmus rubra* and *Hydrastis canadensis*. Knowing slippery elm and goldenseal by their Latin names allowed me to break the language barrier and get the medicines I wanted in my time of need.

Herbal Actions

Again, herbal actions help define herbs by their action in the body. This classification sorts herbs into action groups. Note, however, that blending effective formulas is much more then picking herbs based on their herbal actions. Refer to my book *The Herbal Apothecary* or other resources to understand the dynamics of herbal formulation. The list below is extensive and includes some older terms rarely used today, but they're helpful in preserving the art and science of traditional herbal medicine.

Abortifacient	Herbs that terminate pregnancy or induce premature birth
Acrid	Herbs with a hot, bitter taste or that cause heat and irritation when applied to the skin
Adaptogen	Herbs that increase the body's resistance to biological, emotional, environmental, or physical stressors and promote optimal physiological function
Adjuvant	Herbs added to a mixture to aid the effects of the principal ingredient
Adrenal Tonic	Herbs that improve the tone, histology, and function of the adrenal glands
Alexipharmic	Herbs that ward off disease or the effects of poison
Alterative	Herbs that gradually restore the proper function of the body, usually by improving nutrition and increasing health and vitality
Analgesic	Herbs that reduce or diminish pain

Anaphrodisiac	Herbs that reduce sexual desire or ability
Anesthetic	Herbs that deaden sensation
Anodyne	Herbs that ease or mitigate pain
Antacid	Herbs that counteract or neutralize acidity in the gastrointestinal tract
Anthelmintic	Herbs that expel intestinal worms
Antiallergenic	Herbs that tone down allergic responses, often by stabilizing mast cells
Antiandrogenic	Herbs that inhibit or modify the action of androgens (male sex hormones)
Antianemic	Herbs that prevent or correct anemia
Antiarrhythmic	Herbs that prevent or are effective against arrhythmias (variations from the normal rhythm or rate of the heartbeat)
Antiasthmatic	Herbs that prevent or relieve asthma attacks

Antibacterial	Herbs that inhibit the growth of or destroy bacteria
Antibilious	Herbs that counteract biliousness or excess bile
Antibiotic	Herbs that destroy or arrest the growth of microorganisms
Anticariogenic	Herbs that reduce the incidence of dental caries (tooth decay)
Anticatarrhal	Herbs that help the body remove excess catarrhal buildups from the sinus cavity area or other areas
Anticoagulant	Herbs that prevent clotting in a liquid (i.e., blood)
Anticonvulsant	Herbs that prevent or arrest seizures
Antidepressant	Herbs that alleviate depression
Antidiabetic (Hypoglycemic)	Herbs that alleviate diabetes or symptoms of the disease
Antidiarrheal	Herbs that alleviate diarrhea
Antidotal	Herbs that act as an antidote, counteracting poison or anything noxious
Antiecchymotic	Herbs that prevent bruising
Antiedematous	Herbs that prevent or alleviate edema (fluid retention)

Antiemetic	Herbs that reduce the feeling of nausea and relieve or prevent vomiting
Antifungal	Herbs that destroy or inhibit the growth of fungi
Antihemor-rhagic	Herbs that reduce or stop bleeding when taken internally
Antihydrotic	Herbs that reduce or suppress excessive perspiration
Anti-inflammatory	Herbs that help the body combat inflammation; demulcents and emollient can also act in the same way (see section 29)
Antilithic	Herbs that prevent the formation of stones or gravel in the urinary system, dissolve those already there, and assist with their removal
Antimicrobial	Herbs that help the body to resist or destroy pathogenic microorganisms
Antioxidant	Herbs that protect against oxidation and free radical damage
Antiparisitic	Herbs that inhibit the activity of or kill parasites
Antiperiodic	Herbs that reduce fever
Antiphlogistic	Herbs that reduce inflammation and pain
Antiplatelet	Herbs that reduce platelet aggregation

Antiprostatic	Herbs that reduce symptoms from the prostate gland
Antiprotozoal	Herbs that kill or inhibit the growth or activity of protozoa
Antipsoriatic	Herbs that relieve the symptoms of psoriasis
Antiputrid	Herbs used in states of decay or putrefaction
Antipyretic	Herbs that alleviate fever
Antirheumatic	Herbs that relieve rheumatism
Antiscorbutic	Herbs that prevent scurvy
Antiscrofulous	Herbs that counteract scrofula
Antiseptic	Herbs that prevent putrefaction or infection
Antispasmodic	Herbs that can prevent or ease spasms or cramps in the body
Antithyroid	Herbs that reduce the activity of the thyroid gland
Antitussive	Herbs that relieve amount or severity of coughing
Antitumor	Herbs that have action against malignant tumors
Antiulcer	Herbs that relieve ulceration
Antiviral	Herbs that kill or inhibit the growth of viruses
Anxiolytic	Herbs that alleviate anxiety

Aperient	Herbs that promote a mild movement of the bowels
Aphrodisiac	Herbs that stimulate the sexual organs and excite sexual desire
Appetizing	Herbs that increase the appetite
Aromatic	Herbs with an agreeable odor and stimulating qualities
Astringent	Herbs that contract tissue by precipitating proteins and can thus reduce secretions and discharges; contain tannins
Attenuant	Herbs that attenuate (dilute) humors and secretions
Balsam	A resinous substance obtained from the exudations of various trees and used in medicinal preparations
Bitter	Bitter herbs that stimulate the digestive system through a reflex via the taste buds
Bladder Tonic	Herbs that improve the tone and function of the bladder
Bradycardic	Herbs that act against abnormal slowness of the heartbeat
Bronchospasmolytic	Herbs that reduce spasm in the lower respiratory tract
Calmative	Herbs that have a mild sedating or tranquilizing effect

Cancer Preventative	Herbs that prevent the incidence of cancer
Cardiac	Herbs that affect the heart
Cardio-protective	Herbs that protect cardiac tissue against hypoxia (oxygen deficiency) and decrease the risk of heart damage
Cardiotonic	Herbs that improve the force of contraction of the heart
Carminative	Herbs that prevent the production and facilitate the expulsion of gas in the gastrointestinal tract
Cathartic	Herbs that produce an evacuation of the bowels; laxative
Caustic	Corrosive herbs capable of burning away tissues
Cephalic	Herbs that act remedially on the head for headache
Cholagogue	Herbs that stimulate the release and secretion of bile from the gall bladder into the intestines; have a laxative effect
Choleretic	Herbs that prevent excess bile
Circulatory Stimulant	Herbs that improve blood flow through body tissues
Coagulant	Herbs that induce clotting in a liquid (i.e., blood)
Cognition Enhancing	Herbs that facilitate learning or memory

Cordial	Herbs beneficial to the heart
Corrective	Herbs that assist in restoring the body to a healthy state
Counterirritant	Herbs that produce irritation in one part of the body to counteract irritation or inflammation in another part
Culinary	Herbs used in cooking
Demulcent	Herbs, usually rich in mucilage, that can soothe and protect irritated or inflamed internal tissue, particularly mucous membrane
Deobstruent	Herbs that clear away obstructions by opening the natural passages of the body
Depressant	Herbs that lessen nervous or functional activity; the opposite of a stimulant
Depurative	Herbs used to purify the blood
Dermatic	Herbs that act upon the skin
Detergent	Cleansing herbs
Detersive	Herbs that cleanse ulcers or carry off foul matter
Diaphoretic	Herbs that aid the skin in the elimination of toxins and promote perspiration
Digestive Stimulant	Herbs that stimulate the function of the gastrointestinal organs involved in digestion

Disinfectant	Herbs that cleanse infections by destroying or inhibiting the activity of disease-producing micro-organisms		Female Tonic	Herbs that improve the tone, vigor, and function of the female reproductive system
Diuretic	Herbs that increase and assist with elimination of urine		Galactagogue	Herbs that help stimulate and increase milk flow
Dopamine Agonist	Herbs that bind to and activate dopamine receptors		Gastric Stimulant	Herbs that stimulate the function of the stomach
Ecbolic	Herbs that aid childbirth by increasing uterine contractions		Hemostatic	Herbs that stop bleeding
			Hallucinogen	Herbs that induce hallucinations
Emetic	Herbs that induce vomiting		Hepatic	Herbs that aid, tone, and strengthen the liver, and that increase the flow of bile
Emmenagogue	Herbs that stimulate and normalize menstrual flow; can include herbs that act as tonics on the female reproductive system		Hepatoprotective	Herbs that protect the hepatocytes (liver cells) against toxic damage
Emollient	Herbs that soften, soothe, and protect the skin; act externally as demulcents do internally		Hepatotrophorestorative	Herbs used to restore the integrity of liver tissue
			Hydragogue	Herbs that cause a watery discharge
Estrogen Modulating	Herbs that act subtly to promote estrogen production and effects in the body		Hypertensive	Herbs used to decrease blood pressure
			Hypnotic	Herbs that promote sleep
Exanthematous	Herbs related to skin diseases or eruptions		Hypocholesterolemic	Herbs that reduce the level of cholesterol in the blood
Expectorant	Herbs that assist the body in removing excess mucus from the respiratory system		Hypoglycemic	Herbs that reduce the level of glucose in the blood
			Hypolipidemic	Herbs that reduce the lipid level (cholesterol and tri-glycerides) of the blood
Febrifuge	Herbs that reduce or eliminate fevers		Hypotensive	Herbs that reduce blood pressure

Immune Depressant	Herbs that reduce immune function; used particularly when part of the immune system is overactive
Immune Enhancing	Herbs that enhance immune function
Immune Modulating	Herbs that modulate and balance the activity of the immune system
Insecticidal	Herbs that kill insects
Irritant	Herbs that cause pain or heat
Laxative	Herbs that promote bowel movement and offer relief from constipation
Liniment	A medicine acting as an embrocation (lotion)
Lithotriptic/ Antilithic	Herbs that can crush a calculus (an abnormal con-cretion, usually in the form of mineral salts) within the bladder
Local Anesthetic	A substance that removes sensation or pain when applied locally
Lymphatic	Herbs that assist detoxification by their effect on lymphatic tissue; often also improve immune function
Male Tonic	Herbs that improve the tone, vigor, and function of the male reproductive system
Maturative	Herbs that promote suppuration (pus)

Mucilaginous	Herbs characterized by a gummy or gelatinous consistency
Mucolytic	Herbs that help break up and disperse sticky mucus in the respiratory tract
Mucoprotective	Herbs that protect the mucous membranes, especially in the context of the gastric lining
Mucous Membrane Tonic	Herbs that improve the tone, vigor, and function of the mucous membranes (particularly of the respiratory tract)
Mydriatic	Herbs that dilate the pupil of the eye
Myotic	Herbs causing an unnatural contraction of the pupil of the eye
Narcotic	Herbs that relieve pain and induce sleep when used in medicinal doses; in large doses, can produce convul-sions, coma, or death
Nauseate	Herbs that produce an inclination to vomit
Nephritic	Herbs applicable to diseases of the kidney
Nervine	Herbs that have a beneficial effect—calming, soothing, or strengthening—on the nervous system
Neuro-protective	Herb that helps prevent damage to the brain or spinal cord from ischemia, stroke, convulsions, or trauma

Nutritive	Herbs that nourish the body
Odontalgic	Herbs used for a toothache
Ophthalmic	Herbs used on inflammation of the eye or its appendages
Ovarian Tonic	Herbs used to enhance the tone, vigor, and function of the ovaries
Oxytocic	Herbs that stimulate contractions of the uterus
Parasitic	Herbs that kill parasites
Parturient	Herbs that induce labor and assist in the efficient delivery of the fetus and the placenta
Partus Preparator	Herbs taken in preparation for labor and childbirth (treatment usually begins in the second trimester)
Pectoral	Herbs that strengthen and heal the respiratory system
Peripheral Vasodilator	Herbs that dilate or widen the peripheral blood vessels and thereby improve circulation to the peripheral tissues; may assist in reducing blood pressure
Poison	Herbs that have a harmful or destructive effect when in contact with living tissue
Progestogenic	Herbs that promote the effect or production of progesterone
Prolactin Inhibitor	Herbs that inhibit the secretion of prolactin

Protozoicidal	Herbs that kill protozoa (e.g., amoebae)
Pulmonary	Herbs that strengthen the lungs
Pungent	Hot-tasting herbs that act on a common group of nerve cell receptors, having the effect of warming the body and improving digestion and circulation
Purgative	Herbs that purge the body by emesis or via the bowels
Refrigerant	Herbs that are cooling and/or relieve thirst
Restorative	Herbs that restore consciousness or normal physiological activity
Rubefacient	Herbs that cause redness of the skin when applied topically, helping to increase blood flow and circulation
Sedative	Herbs that calm the nervous system and reduce stress and nervousness
Sexual Tonic	Herbs that improve the tone, vigor, and function of the sexual organs
Sialogogue	Herbs that increase the secretion of the salivary glands
Soporific	Herbs that induce sleep
Spasmolytic	Herbs that reduce or relieve smooth muscle spasm

Specific	Herbs that cure or alleviate a particular condition or disease
Sternutatory	Herbs that provoke sneezing
Stimulant	Herbs that excite or quicken the activity of the physiological process
Stomachic	Herbs that strengthen and stimulate the stomach
Styptic	Herbs that stop bleeding when applied locally
Sudorific	Herbs that produce sweating
Thyroid Stimulant	Herbs that enhance the activity of the thyroid gland
Tissue Perfusion Enhancing	Herbs that enhance the flow of nutrients into a tissue
Tonic	Herbs that strengthen and enliven specific organs or the whole body
Toxic	Herbs of a stimulating, narcotic, or anesthetic nature
TSH Antagonist	Herbs that block the activity of TSH (thyroid stimulating hormone)
Urinary Antiseptic	Herbs that inhibit the growth of or destroy microorganisms within the urinary tract

Urinary Demulcent	Herbs that have a soothing effect on mucous membranes of the urinary tract
Uterine Sedative	Herbs that reduce the activity of the uterus
Uterine Tonic	Herbs that increase the tone of the uterine muscle
Vasoconstrictor	Herbs that constrict or narrow blood vessels
Vasodilator	Herbs that dilate or widen blood vessels
Vasoprotective	Herbs that protect the integrity of the blood vessels
Venotonic	Herbs that improve the tones and function of the veins
Vermicide	Herbs that destroy intestinal worms
Vermifuge	Herbs that expel intestinal worms
Vesicant	Herbs that produce blisters
Vulnerary	Herbs that are applied externally to help heal wounds and cuts
Weight Reducing	Herbs that assist in the reduction of body weight

Herbal Bio Constituents

The rise of ethnopharmacology and pharmacognosy led to the scientific labeling and defining of individual herbs' medicinal parts, called *herbal bio constituents* or *phytochemicals*. Use the information below to build upon your herbal knowledge for more in-depth study of herbal medicine from a scientific perspective.

Alkaloids: Ammonia compounds with nitrogen bases. Alkaloids have strong biological effects. Stimulant, narcotic, and toxic by principle, they are extremely bitter by nature. Often concentrated in the seeds and roots of herbs.

Formulation tips: Tannins precipitate alkaloids, so please keep in mind when formulating. Alcohol soluble, rarely water soluble, and nearly insoluble in fixed oils.

Glycosides: Condensation products of sugars. Although not true herbal bio constituents, glycosides easily bind to carbon, nitrogen, alcohol, or sulfur, turning them into something else, including any of the other bio constituent groups. They are sugars by principle and bitter by nature. Due to its bitter nature, this group is often given to correct digestion and stimulate appetite.

Formulation tips: Alcohol and water soluble.

Phenols: Polyphenol extracts. They work with the defense systems of the body.

Flavonoids: Polyphenol type. Known as antioxidants and free radical scavengers. They tend to give integrity to structures. In plants, they play an important role as growth regulators. They are also known to strive for balance when under attack from such things as allergens, viruses, and other foreign invaders.

Tannins: Polyphenol type with a propensity for acidic reactions. Often used as antiseptics and as healing agents. Think *astringent* when you think of tannins. Used to tighten up vessels, tissues, watery secretions, and the like.

Formulation tips: Alcohol and water soluble.

Saponins: The word is derived from the plant *Saponaria vaccaria*; it describes its soap-like quality when it's mixed with water, producing a lather. Similar in structure to many hormones such as estrogen, progesterone, and cortisol. When considering saponins, one must review their toxic effects. They can at times produce an irritation to the respiratory track, digestive track, or mucous membranes of the body. Due to their hemolytic properties, their ability to rupture cell walls of red blood cells, they should never be used intravenously or intramuscularly, such as in IV therapy or injection.

Formulation tips: Alcohol and water soluble.

Terpenes: These consist of chains of carbon and hydrogen units. They are variable in action, from highly stimulating to deeply sedative. Most of them are highly aromatic; some can be broken down and processed extremely quickly, which can lead to strong effects requiring caution. Antimicrobial by principle.

Formulation tips: Alcohol soluble, insoluble in water.

Volatile oils: Synonymous with essential oils, volatile oils are highly aromatic and typically grouped as antimicrobial by principle. Derived by a steam distillation process, they are very different from a simple herbal oil. Used to stimulate or sedate tissues, they are most often phenolic by principle, but they can also produce some alkaloids.

Formulation tips: Alcohol and oil soluble.

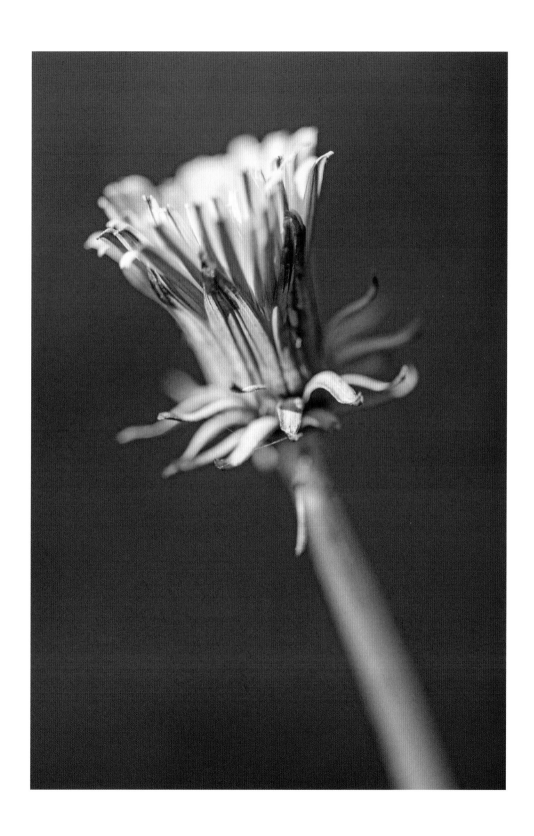

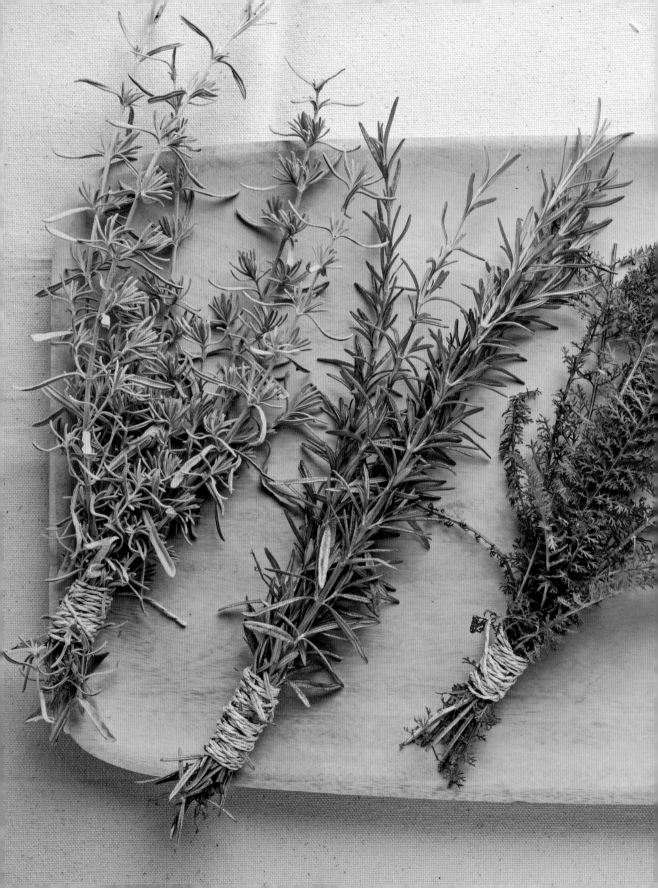

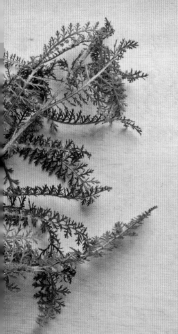

CHAPTER 2

Herbs for Women

THROUGHOUT THE REST OF THIS BOOK, I will be referencing herbs by name. Although many of the herbs listed below are used throughout the body, this materia medica is curated to how these herbs are used for women's health. I say this because it is important not to pigeonhole an herb into one function. The key is to remember that herbs have an affinity for certain areas of the body, but their actions can be applied in many ways. Earlier I mentioned the art of creating a medicinal herb blend verses simply picking herbs based on their action. Although using single herbs for specific reasons has merit, understanding tissue states and herbal energetics is important to creating a successful blend. If you are looking to learn more, refer to the book *The Herbal Apothecary* or other resources on creating medicinal blends. In the meantime, learn the herbs. I suggest getting an ounce (28 g) of one or two herbs to play with each week. Look at them in their fresh or dried form, smell them, and try them as tea or tincture. This will provide a much richer experience versus just reading about them. Be sure to note in your journal how they taste or make you feel. This information will provide you with keen insight into the herb.

Starting Your Herb Journal

An herb journal is an essential part of every herbal enthusiast's journey. It is a place to keep notes and recipes and write down pearls of information to use later. It allows you to reflect your thoughts on how an herb did or didn't work for you, how it made you feel, and specifics for a recipe that you want to duplicate.

This book divides life into three phrases: Dawning, menarche to young adulthood; Living, young adulthood through reproductive years; and Fulfillment, the post-reproductive years. But before we discuss herbs by life phase, this section lists them individually. Each entry includes the herb's name, the phase of life in which it is most often used, its primary use, its herbal action, and foundational information about it. These brief descriptions only provide the tip of the iceberg when it comes to knowing each herb and its potential. Review these first to familiarize yourself and then go to the groupings list. It makes for quick referencing when you are looking things up. I've also included herb lists throughout the book for easy shopping, recipe fulfillment, and/or pantry stocking.

AGRIMONY, *Agrimonia eupatoria*

A. **PHASE OF LIFE**: Dawning

B. **PRIMARY USE**: A friend to those who wear the mask that all is well but are suffering inside

C. **HERBAL ACTION**: Emmenagogue, hepatic, astringent, cholagogue

My first encounter with agrimony, while I was walking through my mentor's garden, was when it literally jumped out and grabbed me. Its little yellow flowers and the stickers that attached themselves to me instantly bedazzled me. I felt calmer just standing next to it. Agrimony is traditionally used to calm digestion, aid in menstrual regulation when menses are present but not consistent, and support the liver-gallbladder connection. But it was the plant's emotional offerings that affected me the most. It's recommended for those who have had a shock or a moment when their experience caused them to hold their breath, and they've been holding it ever since; agrimony reminds us to breathe again. For those who hold everything in their stomach, agrimony aids in the release of tension in the entire abdominal area, including the uterus.

ALFALFA LEAF, *Medicago sativa*

A. **PHASE OF LIFE**: Living

B. **PRIMARY USE**: Support for and an alkalizing effect on the structures of the body

C. **HERBAL ACTION**: Tonic, diuretic

Whenever minerals are needed, I use alfalfa. If I notice prolapse, loose ligaments, or generalized fatigue, I often include alfalfa. Some herbalists believe—and I can't argue—that alfalfa's mineral content fluctuates widely. As with anything, knowing your source is important. But I also can't deny that my goats crave the extra minerals once they are with babe. Currently, I have nine goats, four of whom are pregnant. The smallest of all of them, Electra, grabs three alfalfa flakes each morning and hoards them for herself. If the other goats try to share, she jumps on their back until they finally go away!

Alfalfa also has an alkalizing effect on the body, combating the overly acidic nature of our digestive tracks and other systems that present as irritated.

ANGELICA ROOT, *Angelica archangelica*

A. **PHASE OF LIFE**: Dawning, Living

B. **PRIMARY USE**: Support for the female reproductive system through the movement of blood

C. **HERBAL ACTION**: Emmenagogue, nervine, stimulant, tonic, carminative, bitter

Once coined "the female ginseng," angelica is a superior women's reproductive tonic. It's good for pelvic congestion and suppression of the menstrual cycle. It gently warms the pelvis and moves circulation throughout. Traditionally used for menstrual headaches and premenstrual syndrome (PMS) digestive upset, it's also good to include in menstrual balancing recipes when the liver appears to be a bit sluggish.

ANISE SEED, *Pimpinella anisum*

A. **PHASE OF LIFE**: Fulfillment

B. **PRIMARY USE**: Easing digestion, inhibiting cramping

C. **HERBAL ACTION**: Antispasmodic, aromatic, carminative, digestive, tonic

Anise is best known for its abilities to soothe digestion and gas, but its pain relief goes beyond the digestive track. You can use anise seed oil for menstrual cramping and/or tender breasts. Babies who are suffering from colic will benefit from teaspoon drops of anise seed tea. If taken in larger, concentrated quantities, it may bring on menstruation. Anise water is thought to increase milk production in nursing mothers.

ASHWAGANDHA, *Withania somnifera*

A. **PHASE OF LIFE**: Fulfillment

B. **PRIMARY USE**: A natural brain booster, energizer, and overall tonic for the body

C. **HERBAL ACTION**: Adaptogen, tonic, aphrodisiac, hepatic, sedative

I first began using ashwagnadha as a tonic for a severely immune debilitated patient. Its ability to strengthen the overall immune system as well as bodily systems made it almost seem like a superfood. It also worked on the central nervous system, making the patient less stressed and better able to handle the hurdles her body was presenting. I've recommended it for the two major types of anemia, Pernicious anemia and iron deficiency anemia—not to fill the gap of deficiency but to provide a stabilizing tonic to decrease overall fatigue. Research shows that the amino acids present in ashwagnadha help improve brain function, calm the overly excitable states, and even work to balance natural sleep cycles.

ASTRAGALUS, *Astragalus membranaceus*

- **A. PHASE OF LIFE:** Living, Fulfillment
- **B. PRIMARY USE:** Support for the overall vitality of the immune system
- **C. HERBAL ACTION:** Adaptogen, immunostimulant, antiviral, nervine

Astragalus is another herb that can be taken as medicine or added to your food to turn your culinary creations into medicine. It can often be purchased in whole root form at co-op grocery stores, and it can turn soups into power-packed immune system boosters. Although astragalus will do its best to keep the colds and flus away, its job isn't to help fight them. Instead, it works to tone the overall immune functions of the body, increasing your body's ability to keep invaders from settling in. It also influences the central nervous system, which means it can encourage the reduction of stress. When stress goes down, immune systems strength goes up. As an adaptogen, astragalus finds imbalance in the body and corrects it.

BLACK COHOSH, *Cimicifuga racemose, Syn. Actaea racemose*

- **A. PHASE OF LIFE:** Living, Fulfillment
- **B. PRIMARY USE:** Stimulating labor and regulating contractions
- **C. HERBAL ACTION:** Emmenagogue, antispasmodic, nervine, alterative, expectorant, diuretic

Although we typically think of black cohosh as a women's herb, it should also be considered a powerful normalizer for both men and women to balance hormones and to reduce pain and discomfort. It helps reduce cramping or ovarian pain, quiets the womb (unless it is time for birth), reduces arthritic and nerve pain, and acts as an excellent central nervous system healer. I first used it as an anxiety treatment in 1999 after reading about Michael Tierra's use of it with various nervous conditions with concomitant muscle pain. Michael Tierra is an herbalist who specializes in blending Eastern and Western herbs and has a great herb book called *The Way of the Herbs*. (Side note: His wife, Lesley Tierra, wrote my favorite beginner Chinese herb book called *The Herbs of Life*.) But the nerve tonic Michael wrote about worked well, and I continued to use it in broad ways to reduce muscle tension and tremors caused by stress, menopausal symptoms, anxiety, insomnia, and reproductive congestion.

BLESSED THISTLE, *Cnicus benedictus*

- A. **PHASE OF LIFE**: Living
- B. **PRIMARY USE**: Nutritive, hormone balancing, liver support, pregnancy
- C. **HERBAL ACTION**: Bitter, emmenagogue, galactagogue, stimulant, tonic

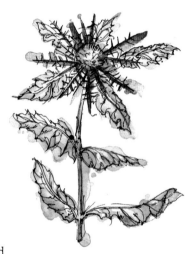

Blessed Thistle

When I think of blessed thistle, I think of hormonal balancing through liver detoxification. But it's actually a multitasker, supporting the endocrine system while aiding the master detoxifying actions of the liver. This herb is a great choice when you suspect that your hormone imbalance is not originating from the reproductive organs themselves. Its ability to gently cleanse the blood makes it helpful for troublesome skin conditions such as acne. Traditionally known as a "corrective" for reproductive systems, it will lower what is too high and raise what is too low. It helps women who have irregular menstrual cycles or who are looking to increase breast milk supply. For those experiencing emotional fluctuations, blessed thistle is known to clear and calm the mind and heart. It's a key herb for the women's home herbal pantry.

BLUEBERRY, *Vaccinium* spp.

- A. **PHASE OF LIFE**: Fulfillment
- B. **PRIMARY USE**: A great source of antioxidants that can be used as a food or dried for winter tea recipes
- C. **HERBAL ACTION**: Antioxidant

Although not always readily available at herb shops, blueberries have their place as a medicinal berry. High in antioxidants, they work to scavenge the body for free radicals, improving skin and cellular integrity. The berries also seem to have an affinity for the eyes and heart, making them a worthwhile addition to microcirculatory-focused herbal blends.

BLUE COHOSH *Caulophyllum thalictroides*

A. PHASE OF LIFE: Living

B. PRIMARY USE: Traditionally used to initiate labor and regulate contractions throughout

C. HERBAL ACTION: Emmenagogue, oxytocic, diaphoretic, diuretic

Often combined with black cohosh and drunk as a tea during the last week of pregnancy, blue cohosh is known to prepare the uterus and body for labor. When labor has gone on long enough, blue cohosh can at times provide relief and completion by supporting the fatigued uterus in regular and strong contractions. Considered a uterine stimulator, blue cohosh is also used to bring on menstruation. Other uses for blue cohosh have included amenorrhea, uterine fibroids, and PMS.

BUCHU *Agathosma betulina* (previously *Barosma betulina*)

A. PHASE OF LIFE: Dawning

B. PRIMARY USE: A superior bladder antiseptic helpful with cystitis, infection, and leucorrhea

C. HERBAL ACTION: Antibacterial, diuretic

Buchu is a good choice as dual action for bladder and vaginal inflammation. It has antibacterial fighting power combined with a soothing action to reduce pain and discomfort. When there is no infection but a constant excessive vaginal discharge, buchu is recommended. I recommend this herb when woman present with "cold kidneys." This presents as lower back pain with vaginal and/or bladder complaints but no infection. In Chinese medicine, we would consider it a kidney deficiency, and one of the ways to treat that is to warm up the kidneys. Using buchu, along with wrapping your torso under your clothes, works to raise the energy and temperature of the kidneys.

BUPLEURUM *Bupleurum falcatum*

A. PHASE OF LIFE: Fulfillment

B. PRIMARY USE: Works directly with the liver to clear estrogen

C. HERBAL ACTION: Hepatic, antiviral, antispasmodic, anti-inflammatory

Working on multiple levels, the Chinese medicine herb bupleurum is a superior women's herb. It helps correct estrogen dominance, which often leads to a reduction in tension. It can relieve pain and correct simple digestive complaints. One of the main medicinal components of bupleurum mimics progesterone. Taken throughout the month, it is known to reduce PMS, particularly anxiety, fatigue, and breast tenderness.

BURDOCK ROOT *Arctium lappa*

A. PHASE OF LIFE: Dawning, Living

B. PRIMARY USE: A superior liver-supporting herb; helpful to "ground" those who are often distracted

C. HERBAL ACTION: Tonic, cholagogue, diuretic

Burdock is a helpful herb for supporting the liver's natural detoxification pathways. It can be eaten as well as taken in herbal medicine forms. My family loves our burdock in stir-fry! As with any liver-supporting herbs, you'll get hormonal support. It's traditionally used during pregnancy as a nutritive and helpful herb to stay vital and well throughout.

BURDOCK SEED *Arctium lappa*

A. PHASE OF LIFE: Dawning

B. PRIMARY USE: Soothes and tones the bladder

C. HERBAL ACTION: Relaxant, demulcent, tonic

Note that we're talking about burdock *seed* here; I like to differentiate it from the root, as it has its own action on the bladder and skin. I have found burdock seed to be helpful when a woman is experiencing bladder urgency, particularly when exacerbated by stress. It seems to give tone to areas that are triggered by overly excited nerves. It's also useful for cystic acne to help to clear the body of the buildup leading to breakouts. It's a good one to include in recipes to gain integrity and smoothness to the skin.

CALENDULA FLOWER *Calendula officinalis*

A. **PHASE OF LIFE:** Living

B. **PRIMARY USE:** Skin healing and health, lymph congestion

C. **HERBAL ACTION:** Antibacterial, antifungal, emmenagogue, astringent, anti-inflammatory

Calendula is said to keep the skin healthy and strong. Typically used in salves for burns, cuts, scrapes, and stings because of its antibacterial properties, it also does an incredible job of pulling tissues back together to expedite healing. Only use calendula when you are ready for a wound to close, because it will work quickly. Sometimes a wound needs to be left open for a while so as to not trap in infection or to heal from the inside out—what is known as healing from the first intention.

Calendula is also a safe and efficient lymphatic system agent. I recommend it if you are fighting off a cold or flu, or if you have chronic lymphatic congestion. It's also a gentle normalizer for the female reproductive system; it can help bring on delayed menstruation, reduce cramping, and reducing bleeding and pelvic congestion.

CALIFORNIA POPPY *Eschscholzia californica*

A. **PHASE OF LIFE:** Fulfillment

B. **PRIMARY USE:** An uplifting, pain-reducing, sedative effect

C. **HERBAL ACTION:** Antispasmodic, relaxant, nervine, sedative

This nervine works on the physical level, directly affecting the mental state into relaxation. When your muscles can release tension, chemicals are released, often allowing the mind to shift into a more peaceful state. California poppy is helpful to take before bed or in extreme states of adrenal activation. It's a good choice when pain is inhibiting the ability to sleep. Note that it is contraindicated with monoamine oxidase (MAO) inhibitors.

California Poppy

CATNIP LEAF *Nepeta cataria*

A. **PHASE OF LIFE:** Dawning

B. **PRIMARY USE:** Has a strong healing effect on the stomach, reducing discomfort, tension, and nourishing deficiency

C. **HERBAL ACTION:** Stomachic, antispasmodic, diaphoretic, carminative

I believe that the stomach is where we hold a lot of what we feel. You can relate if you "feel" your stomach tighten with fear or stress. This is my go-to for stomachaches in teenagers, who tend to feel everything around them. It's a wonderful addition to any tea to soothe and strengthen the stomach and digestive track. It's also a good choice for mild fevers to encourage gentle sweating to reduce the fever.

CAYENNE *Capsicum minimum*

A. **PHASE OF LIFE:** Living, Fulfillment

B. **PRIMARY USE:** Stimulates circulation

C. **HERBAL ACTION:** Stimulant, carminative, anticatarrhal, antimicrobial, rubefacient

Cayenne is an excellent stimulator of the body. I use it to move stagnation when pain is present, to warm up the extremities, and any time the brain needs a bit of a boost in memory or clarity in function. When added to creams or lotions in the right amount, it produces a slight warmth to get the blood moving. It's been used to relieve hoarseness, sore throat, toothache, tonsillitis, fibromyalgia, and arthritis and to increase metabolism. There's no need to be wary of cayenne pepper; as with anything, when used with careful consideration, positive results are possible.

CELERY SEED *Apium graveolens*

A. **PHASE OF LIFE:** Dawning

B. **PRIMARY USE:** Anxiety relief

C. **HERBAL ACTION:** Carminative, sedative

I sort of stumbled onto the effects of this herb, and I've loved it ever since. I once had a patient who was one of the most loving and caring mothers around, but she fretted about her children endlessly. Were they sleeping okay, eating right, engaging with friends enough? You name it, she worried about it. When I have patients with anxiety and worry,

I never downplay the realness of what they are experiencing and know it manifests in physical ways such as insomnia, digestive complaints, headaches, and so on. The trouble was that this patient was also not extremely open to trying new treatment ideas. We talked for quite a while, and then she took out some celery sticks for her kids to snack on. In that moment, I remembered that celery seed had been used for anxiety and stress. I asked her if she was open to trying a celery seed tincture and she agreed. Within three days she e-mailed me to say how much her concern seemed to have quieted down. She felt able to breathe through the flashes of fear she had for her family and was able to identify a more rational view. When celery seed is blended with nervines, it tends to soothe panic and extremely stressful moments in women, especially those who are overly concerned about others and the world and are easily triggered. Combining its sedative effects with carminative actions, you also get the relief of tension held in the abdomen. Considered another micro-traversing herb, it can travel into small spaces to move stagnation and release trapped energies. Note that it is contraindicated in pregnancy.

CHAMOMILE FLOWER *Matricaria recutita*

- A. **PHASE OF LIFE**: Dawning
- B. **PRIMARY USE**: A quiet and gentle nervine that works to balance the central nervous system and hormones
- C. **HERBAL ACTION**: Nervine, carminative, bitter, sedative, anti-inflammatory, antispasmodic, emmenagogue

Chamomile tea is many people's first experience with herbal tea. The delicate flowers have an incredible aroma and, if steeped correctly, a sweet and subtle taste. I love growing chamomile in my garden, but I am lucky if I get six cups of tea from my harvest. Collecting the tiny flowers is laborious but worth it for the fresh tea, a very special treat.

Many years ago, I learned that chamomile can have a hormone balancing effect on the reproductive system. Most often this is used in combination with peppermint, taking one cup of peppermint during the first half of the menstrual cycle and chamomile during the second half. I was experiencing irregular cycles at the time and decided to give this a try. Starting simple is the best way to begin with herbs. Although our society often claims, "Go big or go home," herbs typically work wonders in small ways. Ever since I had success with this simple treatment, I've recommended it, with similar positive results. Chamomile is a great addition to any tea for its flavor and the benefits of soothing both the nervous and digestive systems. But don't steep too long, as bitterness will overtake the tea.

CHICKWEED *Stellaria media*

A. PHASE OF LIFE: Dawning, Living, Fulfillment

B. PRIMARY USE: A cooling herb for both internal and external heat conditions

C. HERBAL ACTION: Carminative, demulcent, expectorant, nutritive

I recommend chickweed for topical heat rashes, boils, and hot wounds to reduce the inflammation, which will often allow other herbs to get in and do their work. Internally, chickweed is cooling to the liver and can help with hot flashes and to balance the hormones. If you're experiencing mastitis, applying a fresh chickweed poultice will often produce relief. Almost any heat condition in the body can benefit from chickweed; it's a must-have for any medicine cabinet. Luckily, it is another one of those "weeds" that proliferates in almost every state.

CHICORY ROOT *Cichorium intybus*

A. PHASE OF LIFE: Fulfillment

B. PRIMARY USE: A natural coffee substitute with the additional benefit of nourishing the liver

C. HERBAL ACTION: Appetizer, cholagogue, digestive, diuretic, tonic

The beautiful blooming of the chicory flower is bittersweet for me. Literally and figuratively! It marks the end of summer, but the dazzling blue is mesmerizing. Although it may seem like yet another herb that balances hormones, and it is, it has a unique flavor all its own. I like to nourish my liver while drinking something that tastes very much like coffee from the deeper flavor perspective. Chicory is moistening by nature, so if there is any heat and/or stagnation occurring in the reproductive glands, it may be a good solution to try.

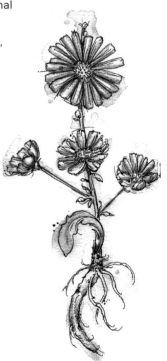

Chicory Root

CINNAMON BARK *Cinnamomum zeylanicum*

- **A. PHASE OF LIFE**: Living, Fulfillment
- **B. PRIMARY USE**: A warming and astringing herb that works to slow or stop bleeding
- **C. HERBAL ACTION**: Analgesic, antibacterial, astringent, antiviral, antioxidant

Research has been done on cinnamon's benefits to both uterine fibroids and polycystic ovary syndrome (PCOS), perhaps due to its warming, stimulating action that moves stagnated energy and blood from the reproductive system. The astringency pulls tissues together and constricts blood vessels to slow excessive bleeding. It is also helpful with leucorrhea.

CLEAVERS *Galium aparine*

- **A. PHASE OF LIFE**: Living
- **B. PRIMARY USE**: A gentle mover of lymphatic fluid to support the immune and kidney systems
- **C. HERBAL ACTION**: Astringent, diuretic, tonic, vulnerary

Cleavers is another one of my favorites from personal use and experience. It seems the lymphatic system is being forced to work harder than ever in our modern world due to environmental exposures. And this herb is always offering itself to help. Growing almost everywhere, it jumps out and clings to us to remind us of its presence. Because it's gentle enough to be used with some regularity, I use it often in my spring cleansing recipes. I've used it with success on lymph congestion throughout the body, including the inguinal glands. It's another herb to consider if you're suffering from acne, to support the waste management of the body.

CRAMPBARK *Viburnum opulus*

- **A. PHASE OF LIFE**: Dawning
- **B. PRIMARY USE**: A go-to herb for menstrual cramp relief that focuses on relaxing smooth muscle
- **C. HERBAL ACTION**: Antispasmodic, astringent, tonic, nervine

Crampbark's effects can often provide relief from acute cramping when one's menstrual cycle kicks in, but I like to recommend taking it before the cycle. Using crampbark as a tonic creates a tonifying effect that can be relaxing to the uterus. This prepares the uterus for menstruation without having to contract so extremely to purge the layers of the endometrium. Herbalist James Duke has cited the two constituents that work to relax the uterine muscles, aesculetin and scopoletin, which have antispasmodic and anodyne properties. Historically, crampbark and its closely related cousin, black haw, have been used to prevent miscarriage by ceasing cramping and helping the uterus relax. They're traditionally combined with astringent and other pain-reducing herbs.

CRANESBILL *Geranium maculatum*

- A. **PHASE OF LIFE**: Fulfillment
- B. **PRIMARY USE**: A powerful astringent to stop bleeding or leucorrhea and balance vaginal pH
- C. **HERBAL ACTION**: Astringent, styptic

When vaginal discharge is excessive, cranesbill can be used internally or externally as a douche. It can also be used as a tincture or tea to inhibit uterine bleeding.

COMFREY LEAF *Symphytum officinale*

- A. **PHASE OF LIFE**: Living
- B. **PRIMARY USE**: Skin healing and health, lymph congestion
- C. **HERBAL ACTION**: Antioxidant, astringent, demulcent, emollient

Comfrey is one of those plants surrounded by controversy. Considered a troublesome weed, this beautiful plant is often ripped from gardens. If people only knew the healing potential it contains! The Latin name comes from the Greek word *symphyo*, meaning "to make grow together," referring to its traditional use of healing fractures. But it also works wonders on the tissues of the body and skin. It has a long history of relieving inflammatory and arthritic pain, as well as just about any skin irritation.

The warnings regarding comfrey began in the 1970s. Experimental data showed that lab rats fed comfrey three to four times their body weight over a long period of time developed liver damage. It would take a human drinking three to four cups of comfrey tea for 140 years to achieve the same effect. Alkaloids known as pyrrolizidines, which are concentrated in the root, less so in the leaves, are the culprits. Extensive research on comfrey and its toxicity potential shows that it's of low toxicity concern.

The absorption of pyrrolizidine alkaloids is limited when applied topically, and the pyrrolizidine alkaloids in comfrey are considered to have a low hepatic toxicity type compared to other types. Check out herbalist Dorena Rode's work if you are looking for more scientific research and information. Comfrey was used and recommended often until the mid-1980s, when unsubstantiated research surfaced. The Henry Doubleday Research Center in England studies a group of people who have been eating comfrey as a cooked green for three generations now, including through pregnancies and lactations; no harm has been reported.

CORN SILK *Zea mays*

- A. **PHASE OF LIFE**: Dawning
- B. **PRIMARY USE**: Soothing irritation and inflammation throughout the body
- C. **HERBAL ACTION**: Demulcent, diuretic

Corn silk is useful in the treatment of painful bladder irritation and for gentle treatment of generalized edema. A demulcent by nature, it helps relieve inflammation in most mucus membranes of the body. This is particularly true in the colon when laxity and irritation have become chronic. Corn silk is known to be helpful in returning tone to this system, as well as to the uterus.

DANDELION *Taraxacum officinale*

- A. **PHASE OF LIFE**: Dawning, Living, Fulfillment
- B. **PRIMARY USE**: Hormonal balancing
- C. **HERBAL ACTION**: Tonic, cholagogue, bitter, stomachic, diuretic

Here's another "weed" that is all around us! You can use all parts of the dandelion plant—roots, leaves, and flowers. The roots act on the liver to gently balance hormones, binding excess hormones and toxins. The leaves work on balancing water states in the body, and the flowers are just for edible fun. Skin also tends to benefit from the regular use of dandelion root and leaf, because it doesn't have to be supporting the liver in detoxification. According to Rosemary Gladstar, the root is invaluable for those going through menopause; it provides the essential nutrients needed to help the hormones find their new level of homeostasis.

DEVIL'S CLAW *Harpagophytum procumbens*

A. **PHASE OF LIFE**: Fulfillment

B. **PRIMARY USE**: Anti-inflammatory actions

C. **HERBAL ACTION**: Anti-inflammatory, bitter, analgesic, anodyne, hepatic

Prized for its herbal constituents, which fight pain and inflammation, initial studies show devil's claw's ability to help with back pain, headaches, and arthritis. It's also traditionally used for gout and digestive complaints, particularly indigestion symptoms.

DONG QUAI *Angelica sinensis*

A. **PHASE OF LIFE**: Living, Fulfillment

B. **PRIMARY USE**: A tonic that works through the liver to balance hormones; also a cardiac tonic

C. **HERBAL ACTION**: Adaptogen, tonic, emmenagogue, hepatic

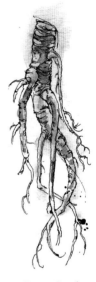

My first experiences with dong quai taught me how nourishing the liver builds healthy blood for the reproductive system. It promotes regular menstruation and tonifies the reproductive system. It has a sweet and spicy taste and can be eaten daily in small amounts for medicinal purposes. When used for the heart, it supports overall circulation and regulates rate and rhythm. Dong quai is also recommended when perimenopause begins to help support the hormones into their new levels. Do not take during menstruation.

Dong Quai

ELEUTHERO ROOT *Eleutherococcus senticosus*

A. **PHASE OF LIFE**: Dawning, Living

B. **PRIMARY USE**: An adaptogen and antiviral herb extraordinaire

C. **HERBAL ACTION**: Adaptogen, antiviral, immunostimulant

Traditionally used mainly as an adaptogen to reduce stress and correct cortisol imbalance, eleuthero also has strong antiviral and immune system fighting powers.

I've always said that when stress goes down, immune function improves. Herpes outbreaks, for example, tend to return when stress is high, almost activating the virus to wake up. Taking eleuthero in advance of stressful times may cut off the reactivation cycle. Eleuthero is also called Siberian ginseng. It does a good job giving strength to the debilitated and weak and those under chronic stress. It has a neutralizing quality, unlike true ginseng, and it does not provoke an overstimulated state.

FENNEL SEED *Foeniculum vulgare*

A. **PHASE OF LIFE**: Living

B. **PRIMARY USE**: Pregnancy, digestion

C. **HERBAL ACTION**: Galactagogue, carminative

This tiny seed is power packed with flavor and healing effects for the body. Used for centuries to heal digestive complaints and regulate the reproduction cycle, it's frequently utilized by most traditional herbalists. Safe enough for children, it is my go-to for my daughter, Cordelia, whenever she is experiencing stomachaches (whether physical or emotional). Fennel works well to release gripping of the abdomen, and new breastfeeding mothers can drink it to help their little ones with colic. It can also be used for morning sickness to calm the queasy stomach and help clear the mind. Modern research shows that it contains some slight estrogenic compounds, which may be why it aids in increasing breastmilk and regulating menstrual cycles. Because of this, avoidance or small doses are necessary for those with estrogen-driven pathologies.

FENUGREEK SEED *Trigonella foenum-graecum*

A. **PHASE OF LIFE**: Living

B. **PRIMARY USE**: Increasing breast milk production, relieving digestive upset and gas

C. **HERBAL ACTION**: Galactagogue, carminative

If you've ever cooked with fenugreek, you are quite familiar with its aroma, produced by the plant's volatile oil. Plants with volatile oils are often soothing to the digestive process, relieving both gas and bloating. There is a reason fenugreek is often included in the rich foods we all enjoy so much!

Fenugreek is one of the most popular herbs for trying to increase breast milk production. Although we still don't have definitive research on how or why it increases breast milk, there is research proving that it does. Research also shows an increase in baby weight and head circumference with the mother's use of fenugreek. One important consideration is dosage; there seems to be agreement that taking less than 3,500 mg, or 3.5 grams, per day will produce no effect. This is an example of needing to take an herb in an adequate dose, repeatedly throughout the day.

Other reported uses include to alleviate heartburn and bad breath, menopause support, and ulcer healing.

GENTIAN *Gentiana lutea*

A. PHASE OF LIFE: Fulfillment

B. PRIMARY USE: A bitters extraordinaire that works to positively promote digestion

C. HERBAL ACTION: Stomachic, carminative, bitter, hepatic

Gentian root is a key ingredient in bitters because it can increase gastric secretions. It promotes overall health of the digestive system and supports the liver by aiding in the breakdown of fat and protein. Bitters are recommended for anyone who feels tired after eating, as they will decrease the digestion time and increase accessible energy from food.

GINGER ROOT *Zingiber officinale*

A. PHASE OF LIFE: Living

B. PRIMARY USE: A warming reproductive tonic, great for relieving congestion

C. HERBAL ACTION: Antispasmodic, carminative, stimulant

I always reach for ginger when I suspect lack of good circulation in the pelvic region. When the vessels surrounding the uterus and ovaries are constricted, you have a lack of warm blood flowing in and around the reproductive system. Using ginger gently warms that up, increasing flow and reducing pelvic congestion. This same effect can be applied to the digestive system, particularly when nausea is present.

GINKGO *Ginkgo biloba*

A. **PHASE OF LIFE**: Dawning, Fulfillment

B. **PRIMARY USE**: Protection for the nerves and cells of the body

C. **HERBAL ACTION**: Antioxidant

Ginkgo is one of the most widely researched herbs, and that research has shown some positive findings. It is well known to provide mental acuity and increased awareness, but new findings are also showing its ability to increase osteoblastogenesis, which is great news for those looking for healthy bone support as we age. As ovulation ceases, it impacts calcium uptake and bone health. Finding ways to keep strong into menopause is vitally important. Although eating the right foods to reach our calcium needs is ideal, it isn't always possible. Another study showed that regular intake of ginkgo helped reduce breast tenderness before menstrual cycles.

Ginkgo

GOAT'S-RUE *Galega officinalis*

A. **PHASE OF LIFE**: Living

B. **PRIMARY USE**: Increasing breast milk production

C. **HERBAL ACTION**: Galactagogue

Goat's-rue is an amazingly supportive herb for all new mothers. I first learned of its use from Juliette de Bairacli Levy, an incredible herbalist from Manchester, England. As an herbalist and veterinarian, Juliette has used her keen sense and knowledge to teach us much about using the same plants that animals use naturally. New goat mothers thrive on goat's-rue, and it has now been proven to increase the natural production of human breast milk. It seems to be particularly helpful for women with low breast glandular tissue, perhaps working specifically on the mammary glands.

Goat's-rue has traditionally been used to treat diabetes; it contains the alkaloid galegine, which has been found to reduce blood sugar and insulin resistance. Some research has focused on goat's-rue's ability to reduce weight.

GOLDENROD LEAF *Solidago virgaurea, Solidago canadensis*

A. **PHASE OF LIFE**: Dawning

B. **PRIMARY USE**: Fighting allergic reactions and improving kidney function

C. **HERBAL ACTION**: Astringent, carminative, diaphoretic, diuretic

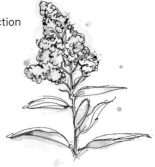

Goldenrod

Goldenrod is often used in bladder tonics or recipes for cystitis. This isn't due to its specific action on the bacterial infection so much as its ability to kick the kidneys into action, increasing filtration and function in an attempt to drive the infection from the body. It is also known to help relieve congestion of the upper respiratory system and combat conjunctivitis.

GOLDENSEAL *Hydrastis canadensis*

A. **PHASE OF LIFE**: Living, Fulfillment

B. **PRIMARY USE**: PCOS, diabetes, digestive healing, infection

C. **HERBAL ACTION**: Antiseptic, astringent, tonic, diuretic

Due to overharvesting, wild goldenseal is nearly nonexistent, and cultivation is a demanding undertaking. Combine these two problems, and you have a very expensive herb. Unfortunately, sometimes goldenseal cannot be replaced with another herb. One such case is extreme digestive damage, when the mucous membranes have lost their integrity and decreased in function. Taking tablespoon doses of goldenseal infusion multiple times per day is incredible treatment. Goldenseal is known to reduce fasting plasma glucose levels, which is great for blood sugar regulation, but also for the benefit of your ovaries, particularly if PCOS is a problem.

GOTU KOLA *Centella asiatica*

A. **PHASE OF LIFE**: Living, Fulfillment

B. **PRIMARY USE**: Well known as a "brain" herb; also supports microcirculation

C. **HERBAL ACTION**: Adaptogen, anti-inflammatory, antimicrobial, vulnerary, vasodilator, astringent, nervine

Gotu kola is a good example of an herb that has been pigeonholed into one action.

When we look deeper into its function, we can see that it has incredible abilities to move stagnation and stimulate healing. It's great for the heart, skin, collagen, and joints. Research shows it may be helpful with pruritic urticarial papules and plaques of pregnancy (PUPPP), endometriosis, and stressful depression.

HAWTHORN BERRY, LEAF, AND FLOWERS

Crataegus oxyacantha, Crataegus monogyna

A. **PHASE OF LIFE**: Fulfillment

B. **PRIMARY USE**: Insomnia, circulation, calming the heart

C. **HERBAL ACTION**: Cardiotonic, astringent, diuretic, hypotensive

One of my favorite herbal combinations for women is hawthorn berry and motherwort. This simple formula connects the heart to the kidneys, offering a rooted foundation upon which to gracefully move through your days. The hawthorn calms and supports the heart physically and emotionally, and the motherwort works to tone the heart and kidneys. Together, a peaceful exchange of energy, like a circuit, is created. I often visualize a kundalini meditation that works to move energy from the root chakra to the head and back to the root. In this mediation you are creating that circuit of energy up, out, and back down again. This is the same cycle I see hawthorn berry and motherwort creating. Meditation in a bottle!

HOP FLOWERS *Humulus lupulus*

A. **PHASE OF LIFE**: Living

B. **PRIMARY USE**: Sleep, stress, breastfeeding, pain relief

C. **HERBAL ACTION**: Bitter, sedative, galactagogue, nervine, anodyne

My mentor, Linda Quintana, and a friend spent a hardworking morning harvesting hops, carrying and filling multiple bags. Then they filled up the car and began to drive home. About fifteen minutes into the drive, Linda looked at her friend, who looked as tired as she felt. All the hops and their pollen had turned the car into a giant sedative capsule, forcing them to pull over and take a long nap in the sunshine. This is how hops seem to work. First you feel good, then hazy, then ready for bed. It's one of my absolute go-to herbs for those struggling with sleep. I also recommend a tincture by the bedside for those who tend to wake up in the middle of the night and have their brains kick on, preventing them from falling back asleep. I also include it in my breastfeeding formulas, as it calms any stress the new mother may be experiencing. It is also a wonderful bitter to support and stimulate the appetite and digestion, as well as a great addition to pain relief formulas.

KAVA *Piper methysticum*

A. **PHASE OF LIFE**: Living, Fulfillment

B. **PRIMARY USE**: Acute stress reduction

C. **HERBAL ACTION**: Sedative, analgesic, diaphoretic, stimulant

Kava has been used for relaxation and sedation for centuries in the tropics, originating in Polynesia. I personally recommend its consumption at home when you have no plans for the evening. Some people are strongly affected by its sedation effects. There have been approximately sixty reports worldwide of kava having toxic effects on the liver, but most of these cases were in combination with either a preexisting liver condition or in those on hepatic medications.

The key to good kava, besides the kava itself, is the preparation. Never use hot water, as higher temperatures destroy kava's active components, kavalactones. Use water or milk at room or lukewarm temperature. A fat-containing liquid such as cow's or coconut milk is best for extraction. Let the kava steep for a few minutes and then strain and enjoy. The longer you allow it to steep, the stronger the effect will be. Some folks recommend putting the kava and milk in a blender and blending for one minute before straining and drinking. Kava has shown promise for anxiety, insomnia, PMS, and menstrual headache relief.

KELP *Ascophyllum nodosum*

A. **PHASE OF LIFE**: Living, Fulfillment

B. **PRIMARY USE**: Nutritive and helpful when working with hypothyroidism, fibrotic breast tissue, PMS

C. **HERBAL ACTION**: Tonic, diuretic

This is another seafood whose nutrients support a multitude of bodily functions. I recommend it for hormonal balancing and fibrotic breast complaints. Kelp doesn't influence the hormones directly, but its nutrients aid in building and processing them. I once recommended a daily dose of dried kelp and almonds to a patient who was having difficulty managing PMS symptoms. Whether the kelp helped or her body worked things out on its own, after two months she reported little to no PMS.

LADY'S MANTLE *Alchemilla vulgaris*

A. **PHASE OF LIFE**: Living, Fulfillment

B. **PRIMARY USE**: Balances and gives tone to the reproductive organs

C. **HERBAL ACTION**: Astringent, tonic, vulnerary, bitter

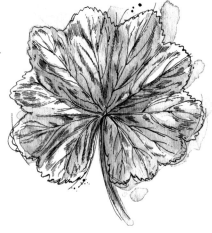

The name says it all! Lady's mantle is a healing ally that seems to be endless in its healing potential. There is little research regarding it, but its historical uses are well documented. Its astringent nature helps to bring tone to the reproductive system, bladder, and pelvic floor. According to Rosemary Gladstar, the women of Switzerland use it to increase the tone of the breasts, a sort of natural breast job. Because of the herbal constituent salicylic acid, it is known to reduce painful menstruation, and the tannins present help with excessive flow. Used during perimenopause, it is used as a tonic to reduce hot flashes and vaginal irritation.

Lady's Mantle

LAVENDER FLOWER *Lavandula officinalis*

A. **PHASE OF LIFE**: Dawning, Living

B. **PRIMARY USE**: Strengthening the wisdom and spirit of every woman

C. **HERBAL ACTION**: Sedative, stimulant, antispasmodic, carminative, tonic

The first herb shop I worked at, Wonderland Tea and Spice, dispensed essential oils per customer request. Naturally, lavender was requested quite often because of its wonderful qualities and common usage, and I cringed each time a customer asked for it. I didn't understand it then, but now I realize some important things about lavender. First, there are many distillations of lavender in essential oil form. The different varieties produce not only very different scents but also actions.

For example, most people consider lavender as a relaxing and calming aroma, but spike, or Portuguese, lavender *Lavandula latifolia* has a much lower linalyl acetate content, making it more stimulating for some. Second, lavender has strong historical connections to encouraging confidence and strength in women. At the time, I was a young woman who was just learning about strength and confidence, perhaps not quite ready for the lessons lavender had to offer. As time went by, however, my connection to it grew, and lavender is now one of my favorite herbs.

LEMON BALM *Melissa officinalis*

A. **PHASE OF LIFE:** Dawning, Living

B. **PRIMARY USE:** A potent nervine that works to support the central nervous system; also often considered for hyperthyroidism

C. **HERBAL ACTION:** Nervine, calmative, emmenagogue, antispasmodic

This unassuming plant works hard in the gentlest of ways. In the Dawning time it helps regulate irregular cycles and ease menstrual cramping. As a nervine, it can be a good choice for young women who are acclimating to living with hormone fluctuations. During pregnancy, it is wonderful as an ice pop to calm nausea or headaches. It is one of the plants that line my front door walkway—its fragrance makes for a wonderful entrance.

LEMONGRASS *Cymbopogon citratus*

A. **PHASE OF LIFE:** Dawning

B. **PRIMARY USE:** Dysmenorrhea, laxity of ligaments

C. **HERBAL ACTION:** Emmenagogue, astringent, nervine, antimicrobial

Lemongrass contains a large volume of volatile oils, which makes it naturally antimicrobial, but let's focus on its ability to reduce painful menstruation. It helps reduce hot stagnated blood that can cause increased cramping during menses.

LICORICE ROOT *Glycyrrhiza glabra*

- **A. PHASE OF LIFE:** Dawning, Living, Fulfillment
- **B. PRIMARY USE:** Often used for fatigue, digestive complaints, hormone regulator
- **C. HERBAL ACTION:** Demulcent, diuretic, expectorant

Licorice has been used to balance women's hormones for centuries. Infertility, menopause, irregular cycles, and high cortisol levels due to stress have all been treated with it. Licorice has estrogenic properties that work to normalize internal hormone levels. I particularly like to use it when there is a digestive complaint in addition to the hormone complaint; it has excellent demulcent properties and works to heal the lining of the stomach as well as the digestive track. It was traditionally used to treat ulcers.

Licorice

A few words of caution: Licorice can be too stimulating for some people suffering from adrenal fatigue. It can feel as though you've drunk too much coffee. For others, it's just the right amount of pick-me-up for the day. Also, licorice has been cautioned against for those with a propensity for high blood pressure and/or water retention. Although it is true that licorice contains compounds that can cause retention of sodium and potassium, fewer than one hundred cases of this effect have been documented worldwide.

MACA ROOT *Lepidium meyenii*

- **A. PHASE OF LIFE:** Fulfillment
- **B. PRIMARY USE:** Hormone balancing, reproductive tonic, stamina
- **C. HERBAL ACTION:** Adaptogen

If stress has taken its toll and you feel fried, maca might be a good fit. If your hormones feel out of balance as well, definitely give it a try. Although it's typically a good choice for hormone regulation, it should be used with caution or not at all by women with estrogen-sensitive conditions. The solid research is still out, but maca may cause some who are genetically predisposed to make more estrogens. When you're entering peri-menopause, your hormones are doing their best to find a new normal, and maca truly helps with the transition on that physical level.

MARSHMALLOW ROOT *Althea officinalis*

- **A. PHASE OF LIFE**: Living, Fulfillment
- **B. PRIMARY USE**: An excellent demulcent promoting anti-inflammatory effects where needed
- **C. HERBAL ACTION**: Demulcent, emollient, diuretic

Marshmallow root is wonderful for any type of irritated tissue, including vaginal. It can be used equally well internally and externally as a wash. It helps with bronchial irritation and with digestive complaints when inflammation is present. Singers can suck on a piece of root for vocal care.

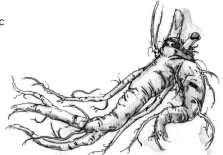

Marshmallow

MILK THISTLE *Silybum marianum*

- **A. PHASE OF LIFE**: Fulfillment
- **B. PRIMARY USE**: A nourishing herb for the liver, with fibroid fighter power as well
- **C. HERBAL ACTION**: Hepatic, tonic, bitter

Milk thistle helps keep the healthy liver cells healthy. Taking it is recommended whenever the liver may be compromised in form or function. It's often paired with burdock. As I've mentioned, liver herbs help to balance hormones and/or bind excess hormones. When hormones are out of balance, new and different things can arise in the body. One of those things may be the manifestation of a benign uterine fibroid. Milk thistle tea has also been used topically for acne vulgaris.

MOTHERWORT *Leonurus cardiaca*

A. **PHASE OF LIFE:** Living, Fulfillment

B. **PRIMARY USE:** A heart protective and harmonizing women's herb for hormone and emotional balancing

C. **HERBAL ACTION:** Antispasmodic, astringent, diaphoretic, nervine, emmenagogue, stimulant, sedative

I grow motherwort all around my home, as it is traditionally known to provide energetic protection to your home and family. Combine the folk knowledge with its medicinal properties, and I am a huge advocate of motherwort. First, it balances the connection between the heart and the kidneys. Kidneys contribute to the function of the heart through blood pressure. On an energetic plane, the kidneys root the heart: When the kidneys are functioning, the heart can relax. It does an excellent job of hormone balancing and of calming moments of PMS tension. Motherwort is nature in perfection, with dualistic abilities allowing it to react as needed in given situations. Having both stimulant and sedative properties, it possesses plant intelligence to respond appropriately to what is needed. It is often given when labor is delayed or menstruation is suppressed.

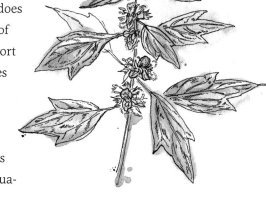

Motherwort

NETTLE LEAF *Urtica dioica*

A. **PHASE OF LIFE:** Living

B. **PRIMARY USE:** Nutritive, allergies, bladder/kidneys, osteoarthritis

C. **HERBAL ACTION:** Tonic, analgesic, diuretic, astringent

Herbalist David Hoffman says, "When in doubt, give nettles." And I agree. This incredible herb has amounts of vitamins and minerals that make it helpful in almost any situation. I include it anytime there is a deficiency picture where trace nutrients and weakness are presenting themselves. If you've yet to harvest nettles in the wild,

I think it is a true rite of passage for any herbal enthusiast. Many don't know, but fresh nettle leaf steamed or sautéed eliminates the stinging effect and creates the taste of springtime for any meal. Their spring arrival is perfect timing alongside the looming allergy season, almost as a reminder to use them during this time. Nettle's anti-inflammatory and histamine reducing capabilities make it the perfect ally for allergy sufferers. With all the B vitamins and trace minerals present, it's no surprise that nettle is great for weakened ligaments and reduced muscle tone. This includes support for both the bladder and the kidneys.

OAT STRAW *Avena sativa*

- A. **PHASE OF LIFE**: Living, Fulfillment
- B. **PRIMARY USE**: Reducing stress and frayed nerve endings
- C. **HERBAL ACTION**: Nervine, tonic, antispasmodic, demulcent

A simple cup of oat straw, or just the milky tops, combined with chamomile is perfect after a day of stress. When we have stressful events and encounters that seem to come out of nowhere, our emotional well-being can feel blindsided. At times like these, look to oat straw. Safe to use when you're pregnant, it can be helpful to use as a douche for the yeast infections that sometimes arise during pregnancy. Because of its high nutritional value, it is valuable not only during pregnancy but also later in life, when calcium and magnesium may be deficient. It's a good herb to use if you are experiencing nervous energy or heart palpitations.

OREGON GRAPE ROOT *Mahonia aquifolium*

- A. **PHASE OF LIFE**: Fulfillment
- B. **PRIMARY USE**: Helpful for the digestive track and liver by working to remove toxins from the body; vaginitis
- C. **HERBAL ACTION**: Diuretic, laxative, tonic

I recommend Oregon grape root as a place to begin for most skin conditions. After four to five weeks of daily intake of tea or tincture, I will reevaluate. Whenever there is constipation, there is often a skin complaint, and Oregon grape root works on both. Although it is listed as a laxative, I have also successfully used it for treating bacterial diarrhea. High in antimicrobial properties, Oregon grape root has been used to treat vaginitis.

PARTRIDGEBERRY *Mitchella repens*

A. **PHASE OF LIFE**: Living

B. **PRIMARY USE**: Hormonal balancing, partus preparator

C. **HERBAL ACTION**: Tonic, astringent, diuretic

Partridgeberry is used for various hormonal imbalances that contribute to irregular cycles, infertility, ovary congestion, or painful menstruation/labor. Traditionally given during the later stages of pregnancy to prepare for a smoother birth experience, it can even be given just at birth to reduce complicating pains. Its astringent nature combined with the hormonal support helps with leucorrhea and prolapse complaints.

PASSIONFLOWER LEAF *Passiflora incarnata*

A. **PHASE OF LIFE**: Living

B. **PRIMARY USE**: A pleasant nervine that works to balance and calm the spirit

C. **HERBAL ACTION**: Nervine, sedative, antispasmodic

Passionflower has long been used to relieve acute stress, such as fear and shock, as well as deficiency that originates out of long-term stress, such as burnout. Try it for insomnia if you tend to overthink every situation. I recommend trying it on its own initially, as it often works well by itself.

PIPSISSEWA *Chimaphila umbellata*

A. **PHASE OF LIFE**: Dawning, Living, Fulfillment

B. **PRIMARY USE**: Bladder tone, membrane protection

C. **HERBAL ACTION**: Astringent, diaphoretic, diuretic, antiseptic

I often include this herb in urinary system recipes when there is infection, prolapse, and lack of tone. Although it is listed as a diuretic, I find it reduces bladder irritation, which often drives urinary frequency and urgency. The natural antiseptic action helps cleanse the bladder system, and it is best drunk as a tea. It's supportive with both urinary and kidney stones, aiding in their breakdown and release through the urinary track.

PLANTAIN LEAF *Plantago major, Plantago lanceolata*

A. **PHASE OF LIFE:** Living

B. **PRIMARY USE:** A powerful drawing and astringent herb for skin and tissues

C. **HERBAL ACTION:** Astringent, demulcent, diuretic, expectorant, hemostatic

Plantain is another herb I use in many cases. Sometimes, when my typical go-tos haven't produced the expected results, I'll add plantain. It's great for the skin and for drawing out toxins from the skin; it also makes a good wash or douche for vaginal discharge. I'll often include it in postpartum teas to aid in the healing process as well as to give tone to the uterus.

POKE ROOT *Phytolacca americana*

A. **PHASE OF LIFE:** Living, Fulfillment

B. **PRIMARY USE:** A stronger lymphatic herb that works to clear congestion from the lymph glands

C. **HERBAL ACTION:** Cathartic, immunostimulant, antibacterial

Poke root works well to relieve congestion of the lymph system. We have lymph glands in our neck, armpits, elbows, chest, breasts, and inguinal areas. All these areas are holding zones for what the lymphatic system collects during the day. When infection or viral load increases, the glands collect a lot and can appear swollen and/ or tender. This is the right time to utilize poke root. I typically use poke root oil on the areas I need, but taking internal doses works well too.

POPLAR BUDS *Populus* spp.

A. **PHASE OF LIFE:** Fulfillment

B. **PRIMARY USE:** Acute muscle discomfort

C. **HERBAL ACTION:** Analgesic, anodyne, anti-inflammatory, antibacterial

Fresh poplar buds contain salicin, which our bodies convert into natural pain-fighting power. It's great for muscle aches and pains; I've also had some success with the topical treatment of rheumatic pains. Apply to the temples or nape of the neck for tension headaches or onto a sunburn for relief and skin healing. It also makes a great addition to healing salves for pain relief, because of its antibacterial effects.

PRICKLY ASH BARK *Zanthoxylum americanum*

A. **PHASE OF LIFE**: Dawning, Living, Fulfillment

B. **PRIMARY USE**: PMS, cramping

C. **HERBAL ACTION**: Anodyne, diaphoretic, irritant, stimulant

It can be virtually impossible to get comfortable when you have severe nerve pain, let alone sleep, work, or exercise. Prickly ash is indicated when the pain is so unbearable you can't get through the day. Its affinity seems to be on nerves, which arise as sharp shooting pains in the body. One patient had menstrual cramping that would shoot pain down her legs, making it almost impossible to walk. Prickly ash provided enough relief that she could move through her days, allowing her to return to school and work.

PSYLLIUM SEED *Plantago ovata*

A. **PHASE OF LIFE**: Living, Fulfillment

B. **PRIMARY USE**: Treating constipation or diarrhea

C. **HERBAL ACTION**: Astringent, laxative, demulcent, antitussive, anodyne

Psyllium can be purchased in the seed powder or husk form and used interchangeably. It's a safe choice for pregnant women who are experiencing constipation or for anyone with digestive issues such as ulcerative colitis or irritable bowel syndrome (IBS).

RED CLOVER *Trifolium pratense*

A. **PHASE OF LIFE**: Living, Fulfillment

B. **PRIMARY USE**: Supporting waste management and reduction of excessive liver by-products

C. **HERBAL ACTION**: Alterative, expectorant, antispasmodic, tonic, estrogenic

Red clover aids in reducing metabolic waste. It works to stimulate anabolic and catabolic reactions and improve overall function, allowing waste to effectively leave the body and nutrients to be preserved. This is why many herbalists call it a blood purifier. It aids the skin for conditions such as eczema. It is also considered helpful for respiratory conditions. Its estrogenic effects can be helpful for soothing menopausal symptoms. See page 159 for more on phytoestrogen and their functions, use, and safety.

RED RASPBERRY LEAF *Rubus idaeus*

A. PHASE OF LIFE: Living

B. PRIMARY USE: Nutritive, pregnancy

C. HERBAL ACTION: Tonic, astringent

Red raspberry is often recommended for use during pregnancy for its ability to strengthen and tone the uterus. It prepares the uterus for labor, giving it strength and endurance capabilities. Regular use is said to prevent miscarriage, encourage progression of labor, and reduce cervical tear potential. I also recommend it post labor to encourage the uterus to return to its normal size and tone, and for anyone experiencing prolapse, the slipping down or forward of the bladder or uterus. Red raspberry leaves contain magnesium, potassium, phosphorus, and vitamins A, C, E, and B complex. It also contains easily assimilated calcium and iron. Another tonic herb, it works to support the ligaments and cartilage of the body. The skin loves red raspberry. Adding it to any facial steam or lotion gives the skin a healthy glow and tighter appearance.

RHODIOLA BARK *Rhodiola rosea*

A. PHASE OF LIFE: Living

B. PRIMARY USE: Any type of chronic stress, cortisol imbalance, or adrenal fatigue

C. HERBAL ACTION: Adaptogen, antidepressant, immunostimulant, aphrodisiac

When a patient presents with adrenal insufficiency or fatigue, I consistently reach for rhodiola. It's a gentle healer of stress, helping to reestablish normal adrenal function versus overstimulation or hyperreaction. I consider the latter a trauma response that has been experienced over and over, cementing a pattern of physical response. For example: If you have a cantankerous relationship with someone in your life, you begin to physically react in the same way each time you interact with this person. Most likely, you'll begin to have a sympathetic response. Your heart rate increases, your digestion system shuts down, and your breathing increases. When you experience this repeatedly, the body is basically preparing for fight or flight. Now, let's say many years go by; the person is no longer in your life, yet you are experiencing the same type of reaction at moments of tiny stressors. You are basically living in the trauma zone, and your body is too. Healing this physically as well as mentally is necessary, and rhodiola can help.

ROSE PETALS *Rosa gallica var. officinalis*

A. **PHASE OF LIFE:** When *aren't* roses a good idea?

B. **PRIMARY USE:** To calm any situation, physical or mental

C. **HERBAL ACTION:** Aperient, astringent, stomachic

What do you think of when you see or smell a rose? Although it may appear delicate, the rose has powerful capabilities to stop bleeding, ease headaches, calm an agitated state, and reduce tension. The rosehips that remain on the bush after the petals fall off make a wonderful addition to flavorful teas, and they are extremely high in vitamin C. A cup of rosehip tea is known to decrease dizziness and ease the stomach. Before I gave birth, I'd heard that rose petals were a strong hemostatic that could be used post labor. The thought of it entranced me, and I tried it. I collected fresh rose petals and wrapped them in cheesecloth. When I was ready, I warmed the wrap in hot water, wrung it out, and applied it like you would a menstrual pad. The soothing was incredible, and my bleeding stopped within the day.

SAGE *Salvia officinalis*

A. **PHASE OF LIFE:** Fulfillment

B. **PRIMARY USE:** Balances hormones, antimicrobial

C. **HERBAL ACTION:** Antibacterial, antioxidant, aromatic, nervine, emmenagogue, astringent

An abundance of medicine from a common garden plant! Every garden should contain sage. It's a historical herb that can be seen in drawings and has been recorded in texts for centuries. Traditionally used for colds and flu, drawing upon its antibacterial powers, it also makes a germ-fighting, throat-soothing gargle. It is unfortunate that the use of sage in the kitchen seems to have declined, as it is another opportunity to bring herbal medicine into everyday cooking. We seem to save it only for the big Thanksgiving dinner;

Sage

yet added to soups and dishes in small quantities, it harmonizes flavors. I was recently at a women's retreat in Hawaii, and my host was making a beautiful purple potato and vegetable soup. I was so happy when she added fresh sage! It, along with a few other herbs, created a beautifully balanced flavor. Sage is often used heavy-handedly in the kitchen, which tends to turn people off. Try experimenting with this easily grown herb to create a new twist to old dishes. From the medicinal perspective, we also use sage for excessive heat, sweating, and uterine bleeding. It's a great addition to your body care products, as it helps combat external odor and can darken gray hair.

SASSAFRAS *Sassafras albidum*

A. **PHASE OF LIFE**: Dawning

B. **PRIMARY USE**: Acne formulas

C. **HERBAL ACTION**: Antiseptic, diaphoretic, stimulant

Known as a good blood purifier, sassafras can be helpful with most skin conditions: acne, eczema, psoriasis, and even gout.

SAW PALMETTO BERRY *Serenoa serrulata*

A. **PHASE OF LIFE**: Dawning

B. **PRIMARY USE**: Affinity for the reproductive system; provides overall tone and support in function

C. **HERBAL ACTION**: Hormone balancing, antiseptic, diuretic

Saw palmetto has largely been marketed to men for prostate health, but it also has great value to the female reproductive system. It's proven to reduce ovarian enlargement with chronic irritation felt in the manner of dull and aching pain. When the ovaries are congested or inflamed, saw palmetto overcomes the irritated conditions and acts as a mild sedative to the ovaries themselves. It can affect the breast tissue, particularly when it is slow to develop or exaggeratedly small. It has been reported to improve fertility and overall tone of the bladder. I use it in many of my skin formulas because it has a relationship with the skin via the liver, often aiding in stubborn acne conditions.

SCHIZANDRA *Schisandra chinensis*

A. PHASE OF LIFE: Living

B. PRIMARY USE: Stress, adrenal support, brain stimulant

C. HERBAL ACTION: Adaptogen, antibacterial

When you read about schizandra, also spelled schisandra, it's hard not to decide that everyone should be using it. It is known to increase energy, slow the aging process, increase mental function, reduce stress, and prolong life. I use it most often for those experiencing long-term mental and emotional stress that has resulted in adrenal fatigue. If you've been dealing with a negative situation in your life for longer than a year, it

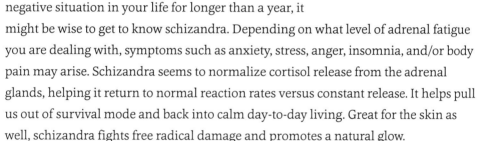

Schizandra

might be wise to get to know schizandra. Depending on what level of adrenal fatigue you are dealing with, symptoms such as anxiety, stress, anger, insomnia, and/or body pain may arise. Schizandra seems to normalize cortisol release from the adrenal glands, helping it return to normal reaction rates versus constant release. It helps pull us out of survival mode and back into calm day-to-day living. Great for the skin as well, schizandra fights free radical damage and promotes a natural glow.

SENNA LEAF *Cassia marilandica*

A. PHASE OF LIFE: Fulfillment

B. PRIMARY USE: A stronger bowel stimulant for constipation

C. HERBAL ACTION: Cathartic, diuretic, purgative

Purgatives by nature tend to cause gripping pains in the digestive track; therefore, I recommend combining senna leaf with aloe or fennel.

SHATAVARI *Asparagus racemosus*

A. **PHASE OF LIFE:** Living, Fulfillment

B. **PRIMARY USE:** A wonderful reproductive herbal tonic for women of any age

C. **HERBAL ACTION:** Tonic, aphrodisiac, galactagogue, antispasmodic, demulcent

An ayurvedic herb, shatavari has made it into the mainstream here in the United States. I recommend it anytime a woman shows general deficiency in her reproductive system. That includes infertility, irregular ovulation/cycles, and low libido at any age. It's also called "She who has one hundred husbands," meaning it inspires the desire for enough action that it would take one hundred men to satisfy it. It is also known to balance the pH of the vaginal track to treat leucorrhea and vaginal dryness and is often used for hot flashes.

SHEPHERD'S PURSE *Capsella bursa-pastoris*

A. **PHASE OF LIFE:** Living, Fulfillment

B. **PRIMARY USE:** Stopping heavy menstrual flow by constricting the uterine vessels

C. **HERBAL ACTION:** Styptic, vasoconstrictor

Shepherd's purse is a high oxytocin that is a strong uterine contractor. It can be used prior to menstruation to help decrease the flow or during active bleeding when bleeding is excessive. Another use is after childbirth if there is too much blood loss. It can be drunk in small doses, 4 to 6 ounces (120 to 175 ml), several times per day, or 2 dropperfuls ever hour or so until bleeding slows or stops.

SKULLCAP *Scutellaria lateriflora*

A. **PHASE OF LIFE:** Living, Fulfillment

B. **PRIMARY USE:** A nervine that targets anxiety and overly high expectations of oneself

C. **HERBAL ACTION:** Nervine, antispasmodic, tonic, sedative

I've coined the term "monkey mind" for the ideal usage of skullcap. Monkey mind happens right as you lie down at night and begin to think about all the things you should have done that day, all the things you shouldn't have done, and all the things you have to do tomorrow. It's your mind pinging from here to there, having difficulty calming down. I also like to use skullcap on those who suffer from internal anxiety. They may look just fine on the outside, but on the inside there is true suffering that needs tending.

SLIPPERY ELM BARK *Ulmus rubra*

- A. **PHASE OF LIFE:** Living, Fulfillment
- B. **PRIMARY USE:** Digestive support to gently move waste throughout the entire intestinal system, bladder tonic
- C. **HERBAL ACTION:** Demulcent, diuretic, emollient, laxative

Anytime digestion isn't working properly, there's possibility for toxic buildup. Chronic digestion complaints not only inhibit nutrient uptake but eventually take a toll on the liver as waste remains in the body longer than it should. Slippery elm bark is a gentle laxative to encourage peristalsis and movement of waste from the body. Anytime bladder irritation is present, drinking slippery elm tea may provide relief due to its emollient action. A wonderful poultice herb, it can also relieve inflammation and pain from most wounds.

SPIRULINA *Arthrospira platensis*

- A. **PHASE OF LIFE:** Living, Fulfillment
- B. **PRIMARY USE:** Nutritive, restorative, and detoxifying properties
- C. **HERBAL ACTION:** Tonic, immune-stimulant, antioxidant

If you could only eat one thing, it should be ocean plants. Packed with amino acids, protein, vitamins, and trace minerals, they are almost a complete food. Now imagine offering that to your body on a regular basis. I've seen hair, skin, and reproductive systems restored when spirulina is included in the treatment regime. It is known to increase metabolism and help the body reduce overall toxic load, which leads to better-looking skin and longevity. It also helps the brain and central nervous system in ways that seem to promote a sense of calm and uplift the depressed spirit.

ST. JOHN'S WORT *Hypericum perforatum*

A. **PHASE OF LIFE:** Dawning, Living, Fulfillment

B. **PRIMARY USE:** Soothing nerve pain, mood stabilizer

C. **HERBAL ACTION:** Nervine, antispasmodic, astringent

Although much of the modern research and marketing of St. John's wort has focused on its ability to relieve depression and sadness, its traditional use is for pain. It's most notable for its ability to ease neuralgia. I've used it for menstrual pain, stomachaches, headaches, and even bronchial irritation, St. John's wort calming each in turn. I have also successfully used it for those suffering from cyclic hormonal depression.

TURMERIC ROOT *Curcuma longa*

A. **PHASE OF LIFE:** Fulfillment

B. **PRIMARY USE:** Reducing inflammation throughout the body

C. **HERBAL ACTION:** Anti-inflammatory, antibacterial, hepatic, analgesic, cholagogue

It seems not so long ago that Americans caught wind of the benefits of turmeric, but ayurvedic medicine has known about them for centuries. This cooking spice has big effects on aches, pain, and inflammation. Turmeric has shown positive results in clinical studies for acute joint or muscle pain and rheumatoid arthritis. It also naturally supports liver and gallbladder functions, aiding in bile breakdown. It's good to consider if prostaglandins are high and causing painful PMS symptoms or cramping.

UVA URSI *Arctostaphylos uva-ursi*

A. **PHASE OF LIFE:** Dawning

B. **PRIMARY USE:** A herb with an affinity for the bladder and kidney systems, focusing on removing stones and infection

C. **HERBAL ACTION:** Antilithic, astringent, diuretic

Also referred to as bearberry, this herb has a stronger effect on the bladder and kidneys than pipsissewa (see page 65) and should not be used long term. Effective with most cases of cystitis and

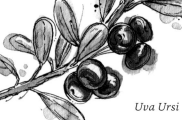

Uva Ursi

stones, it helps rid the body of stones while aiding in pain relief. Topical application is also used to relieve vaginal irritation and pain.

VITEX (CHASTE TREE) BERRY *Vitex agnus-castus*

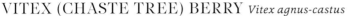

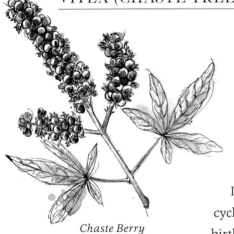

Chaste Berry

A. **PHASE OF LIFE**: Dawning, Living

B. **PRIMARY USE**: *The* herb for estrogen/progesterone balancing

C. **HERBAL ACTION**: Tonic, emmenagogue, adaptogen

When you hear a good quote, it's hard to forget it. Regarding vitex, herbalist David Hoffman once said, "Vitex will always enable what is appropriate to occur." I have found that to be true. Used for normalizing cycles, it also aids in the transition after a woman stops birth control. Endometriosis patients have had some success with pain reduction using vitex, and new mothers have used it to increase breast milk supply. Known to increase progesterone, it can harmonize hormones and circulate the energy of the reproductive system. In traditional Chinese medicine, it is known to possess both warming and cooling natures.

WHITE PEONY *Paeonia albiflora*

A. **PHASE OF LIFE**: Living

B. **PRIMARY USE**: Used when infertility is a concern due to PCOS, endometriosis, ovarian issues, or hormone imbalance

C. **HERBAL ACTION**: Emmenagogue, anti-inflammatory, antispasmodic

White peony is traditionally use in Chinese herbal medicine, but it has made its way into the Western herbal culture over the past few decades. It's a useful consideration when working with ovarian failure or PCOS, as it appears to stimulate the ovarian follicles. Other studies have shown that it positively affects low progesterone levels and regulates estrogen in the body. When used in combination with other emmenagogues, white peony has shown value in bringing on menstrual cycles.

WILD YAM *Dioscorea villosa*

A. **PHASE OF LIFE**: Living, Fulfillment

B. **PRIMARY USE**: The original birth control, wild yam's constituents were the first ingredients used to make contraceptive medications.

C. **HERBAL ACTION**: Antispasmodic, cholagogue, hepatic, anti-inflammatory, diaphoretic, uterine tonic

Wild yam does not contain progesterone, but it does have a precursor that can act as a stimulator to produce natural progesterone. Hence the abundance of wild yam creams on the market. As with any herb, it is important to understand how it truly works in the body so that you can make wise decisions regarding your health care. Wild yam has traditionally been used as a tonic for the uterus and hormones, often leading to a decrease in PMS and uterine cramping. If excess estrogen is a problem, wild yam may be a good herb to try. It's a good one to add to formulas when trying to reduce fibroids. Continuous use for 6 to 12 weeks before steady changes are observed is typical.

YELLOW DOCK *Rumex crispus*

A. **PHASE OF LIFE**: Dawning, Living, Fulfillment

B. **PRIMARY USE**: A liver tonic and herb that helps the body assimilate minerals such as iron more efficiently

C. **HERBAL ACTION**: Antioxidant, hepatic, bitter, astringent

Although not having a high iron content itself, yellow dock can help women assimilate iron in a better way. Iron is typically absorbed in the duodenum, so ensuring digestion is functioning properly and that digestive inflammation is low or absent are key to better iron absorption, as is decreasing excessive bleeding. Therefore, combining carminatives, digestives, and herbs such as shepherd's purse, to decrease menstrual bleeding, should all help increase iron. I often use yellow dock with other hormone-balancing herbs when fibroids or ovarian cysts are present. Yellow dock's affinity for the liver makes it a great addition to skin formulas as well.

YUCCA *Yucca* spp.

A. PHASE OF LIFE: Fulfillment

B. PRIMARY USE: Decreasing inflammation in the body

C. HERBAL ACTION: Analgesic, anti-inflammatory, antirheumatic

There was a yucca plant growing in the backyard of a house I once rented. Knowing its potent anti-inflammatory powers, I was excited about it. Unfortunately, it was growing in the worst place—right along the edge of my backyard sitting space—and after the fiftieth time I got poked and scratched, our relationship began to deteriorate. I resolved that if I couldn't live with it, I'd make the best medicine I could from it. What a torturous endeavor taking out a yucca plant turned out to be! After several days of trying, I still couldn't get all the root base out of the ground. Just like the liver regenerates itself, this thing grew completely back within the year. I made medicine with what I had collected and vowed to honor the plant moving forward. But on my journey, I got to see the freshly cut root and how it wove itself together, just like the body's cartilage and ligaments. Another herb had "shown" me its function in reducing inflammation and stimulating the healing of the fine and delicate structure supporters of the human body.

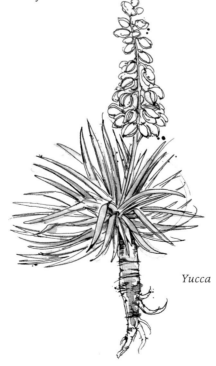

Yucca

CONDITION	HERBS TO TRY
LIFE PHASE: DAWNING	
Regulating cycles	Vitex Berry, Dong Quai, Motherwort, Partridgeberry, Lady's Mantle, Angelica Root, Chamomile Flowers
Painful Menstruation	Crampbark, Silk Tassel, Black Cohosh, Hops, White Oak Bark, California Poppy, Wild Yam, Valerian Root
Spotting Between Periods	Red Raspberry, Vitex, Shatavari, Shepherd's Purse, Chamomile, Lady's Mantle
Breast Tenderness	Turmeric Root, Poke Root, Cleavers, Dandelion Leaf, Lemon Balm, Boswellia
Bloating	Calamus Root, Dandelion Leaf/Root, Fennel Seed, Peppermint, Caraway, Anise Seed, Ginger Root, Chamomile Flowers
Hormone Tonics	Blue Vervain, Burdock, Bupleurum Root, Vitex Berry, Tribulus, Barberry, Maca
Headaches	White Willow Bark, Lavender Flowers, Peppermint, Hops, Blessed Thistle Leaf, Black Cohosh, Turmeric Root, Valerian
Mood Swings	Passionflower, Ginkgo Leaf, St. John's Wort, Chamomile Flowers, Wood Betony, Skullcap, Schizandra Berry
Yeast Infections	Goldenseal Root, Myrrh, Slippery Elm Bark, Usnea Lichen, Pau D'Arco, Yarrow Flower, Lavender Flower, Calendula, Chickweed, Plantain, Comfrey Leaf, Rose Petals
LIFE PHASE: LIVING	
Fibroids	Burdock Root, Dandelion Root, Yellow Dock Root, Oregon Grape Root, Wild Yam Root, Black Cohosh
Ovarian Cysts	Vitex Berry, Blue Cohosh Root, White Peony Root, Chickweed, Crampbark, Poke Root, Nettle Leaf
PCOS	Prickly Ash Bark, Milk Thistle, Dong Quai, Motherwort, Dandelion Root, St. John's Wort, Poplar Buds, Turmeric Root, Saw Palmetto
Endometriosis	Shepherd's Purse, Cinnamon Bark, Blue Cohosh, Cayenne, Mistletoe, Ginger Root

Heavy Bleeding (Menorrhagia)	Shepherd's Purse, Cinnamon Bark, Blue Cohosh, Cayenne, Mistletoe, Ginger Root
Fertility	Maca Root, Spirulina, Kelp, Burdock, Wild Yam, Sassafras, Angelica Root, Sassafras Bark, Black Cohosh, Maca, Dong Quai, Skullcap, Passionflower
Pregnancy	Red Raspberry Leaf, Rose Petals, Partridgeberry, Ginger Root, Lemongrass, Catnip, Nettle Leaf, Lemon Balm, Ashwagnadha Root, Calendula Flowers, Jasmine Flowers
Postpartum	Comfrey Leaf, Calendula Flower, Basil Leaf, Holy Basil Leaf, Rose Petals, Rosemary Leaf, Lavender, St. John's Wort, Astragalus Root, Schizandra Berry, Nettle Leaf, Goat's-Rue, Fennel Seed, Shatavari, Hops, Fenugreek Seed, Red Raspberry Leaf, Blessed Thistle, Oat Straw, Skullcap

LIFE PHASE: FULFILLMENT

Vagina Health	Calendula Flower, Chamomile Flower, Comfrey Leaf, Elderflower
Libido	Shatavari Root, Maca Root, Tribulus, Licorice, Passionflower, Damiana Leaf, Ashwagandha Root, Vanilla Bean, Ginger Root, Cardamom, Rose Petals, California Poppy, Kava Root
Hormone Regulation	Sage, Black Cohosh, Shatavari, Peppermint, Wild Yam, Maca, Black Cohosh, Nettle Leaf, Dong Quai, Yellow Dock Root, Partridgeberry, Vitex Berry, Spirulina, Eleuthero Root, Lemon Balm, Rhodiola Root Bark
Bone Health	Nettle Leaf, Alfalfa Leaf, Comfrey Leaf, Horsetail Leaf, Hawthorn Berry, St. John's Wort, Black Cohosh Root, Yellow Dock Root, Chickweed Leaf, Rosehip Powder, Green Tea Leaves, Dandelion Leaf, Rosehips
Hot Flashes	Black Cohosh, Sage Leaf, Peppermint Leaf, Maca Root, Gingko Leaf, Shatavari Root, Hibiscus, Linden Leaf and Flower, Borage Leaf, Rosemary, Lavender, Yarrow Flowers, Peppermint, Bupleurum Root, Borage Leaf, Chickweed, Cleavers, Burdock Root
Sleep and Stress	Lemon Balm, Chamomile Flower, Wood Betony, St. John's Wort, Angelica Root, Eleuthero Root, Spirulina, Wild Yam, Skullcap, Hawthorn Leaf and Flower, Sage Leaf, Turmeric Root, Sage Leaf, Chickweed, Skullcap
Brain Support	Gotu Kola Leaf, Skullcap Leaf, Linden Leaf, Rosemary Leaf, Sage Leaf, Rooibos, Turmeric Root, Cayenne, Dandelion Root, Nettle Leaf, Licorice Root, Ginkgo Leaf, Hawthorn Leaf and Flower, Lobelia
Thinning Hair	Spirulina, Schizandra Berry, Horsetail, Nettle Leaf, Kelp, Reishi Mushroom, Green Tea, Ginkgo Leaf, Rosemary Leaf

Liver Balancing	Dandelion Root, Milk Thistle, Chicory Root, Burdock Root, Red Clover Blossoms, White Oak Bark, Milk Thistle Seeds, Dong Quai Root, Nettle Leaf, Artichoke Leaf, Yellow Dock Root, Saw Palmetto Berry, Wild Yam Root, Bupleurum, Black Cohosh Root
Digestive Support	Gentian Root, Skullcap Leaf, Ginger Root, Chamomile Flower, Fennel Seed, Anise Seed, Fenugreek Seed, Catnip Leaf, Marshmallow Root, Licorice Root, Cranesbill Root, Goldenseal Root, Plantain Leaf, Oregon Grape Root, Agrimony Leaf, Lemongrass, Senna Leaf, Slippery Elm Bark, Angelica Root
Breast Health	Poke Root, Chamomile Flowers, Dandelion Root, Calendula Flowers, Rose Petals, Comfrey Leaf, Elderberry Flowers
Stress Support	Rhodiola Bark, Schizandra Berry, Ashwagandha Root, Burdock Root, Eleuthero Root, Licorice Root, Passionflower Leaf, Skullcap Leaf, Chamomile Flowers, Catnip Leaf, Lavender Flower, Rose Petals, Celery Seed, Kava Root, California Poppy Flowers, Hops, Agrimony Leaf, Oat Straw and/or Milky Oat Tops, Lemon Balm Leaf, Hawthorn Berry
Bladder Health	Buchu, Nettle Leaf and Root, Red Raspberry Leaf, Fenugreek, Burdock Seed, Lady's Mantle, Goldenrod, Catnips Leaf, Pipsissewa Leaf, Corn Silk, Dandelion Leaf, Cleavers, Marshmallow Root, Chickweed, Chamomile Flowers, Uva Ursi Leaf, Goldenseal Root, Oregon Grape Root
Thyroid Support	Kelp, Parsley Leaf, Barberry, Cleavers, Motherwort, Goldenseal Root, Bugleweed Herbs, Black Walnut Hull, Lemon Balm Leaf, Mullein Leaf, Lobelia Leaf, Spirulina, Eleuthero Root, Alfalfa Leaf, Nettle Leaf, Licorice Root
Cardiac Health	Motherwort Leaf, Hawthorn Berry, Hawthorn Leaf And Flower, Ginger, Hibiscus, Rosehips, Safflower, Gingko Leaf, Maca, Skullcap Leaf, Chamomile Flower, Catnip Leaf, Wild Cherry Bark

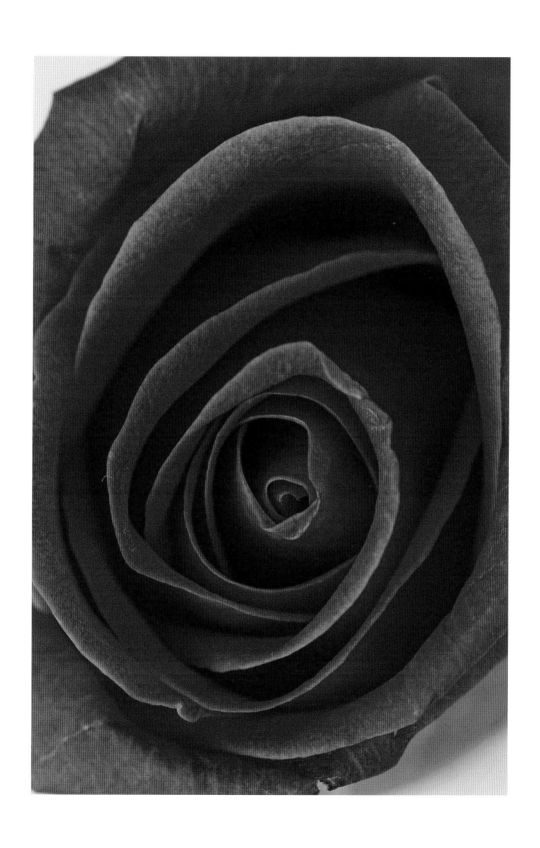

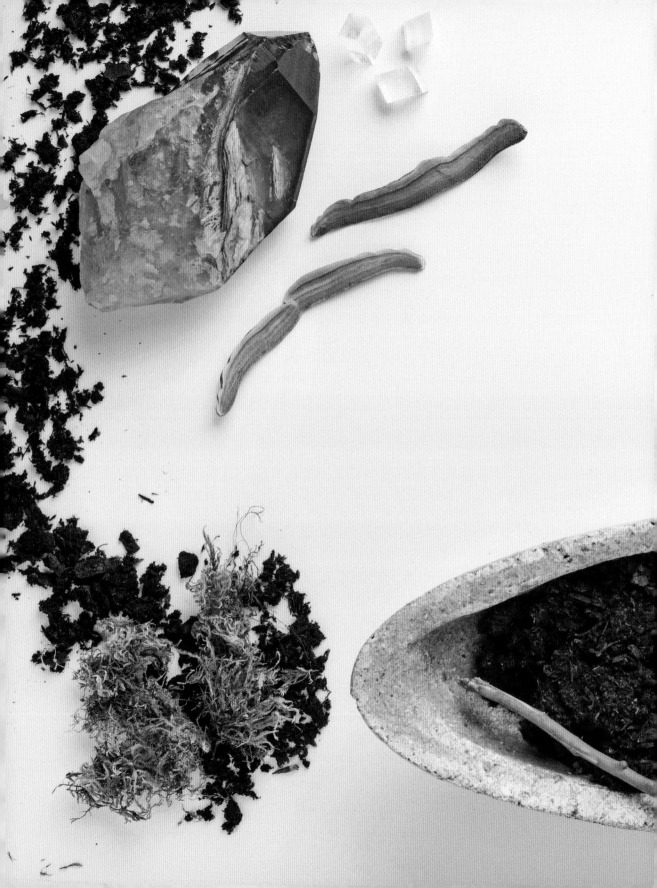

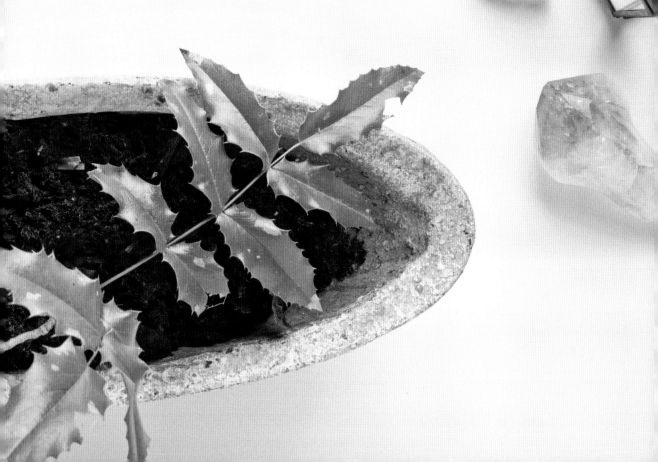

CHAPTER 3

Dawning
Menarche to Twenties

DAWNING is the time before your first menses, menarche, and into your twenties. Your life is dawning like a new day, and you are beginning to awaken to many new and exciting experiences.

Understanding and knowing our female bodies can create deeper connections to ourselves and to those around us. It gives us confidence, which helps us move through our lives prepared and knowledgeable of how to care for ourselves and others. Having positive conversations about menstruation and our fantastic form is vital for healthy self-esteem and confidence. But ask most American girls between the ages of twelve and eighteen about their menstrual cycles, and they'll blush and not want to talk about it. A sense of embarrassment, shame, and sometimes disgust surrounds the natural cycle of the reproductive system. It's too bad because, as women, we contain fascination and power. Imagine if every girl was first told about her reproductive power in a positive, forward manner!

I was a single mom for the first three years of my daughter's life, so everywhere I went, she went. This led to an early introduction to the menstrual cycle for her! Little did I know, but the respect I showed my body during my menses was demonstrating a powerful message to her. I did the best I could to be open and honest while keeping in mind that I was speaking to a toddler. I saw no need to disguise body parts with cutesy euphemisms, nor did I ever try to hide my menses from her when she burst through the bathroom door, as toddlers do. Realizing that someday she too would menstruate, I decided to approach it honestly, directly, and with as much respect and amazement as I could. I shared that our bodies have a unique power that only girls and women have: a uterus. I told her that the uterus is a soft but extremely strong muscle as I did my best to flex my arm muscles. I shared that in many cultures and traditions around the world, the uterus is considered the most special human body part to have. I cupped my hands together into a pod shape and demonstrated how each month the pod grew. Then I shared the ultimate secret—where babies come from, and why the pod grows and shrinks each month, unless a baby is coming.

I cherish the continuous dialogue I have with my daughter through the years, with new and more in-depth information as her body and mind grow. I want to rewrite our youths' relationship with the female body and the menstrual cycle. Many women have created menstrual initiation ceremonies, celebrations, or special activities for girls before and for when they reach menarche. This is a beautiful way to transmit the wisdom of womanhood and bring positive intention into the feminine world.

There are hundreds of positive ways to introduce a young girl to her reproductive life; I encourage everyone to try anything but the hushed tones, tidbits, and fearful sound-bites most children receive regarding the initiation of the menstrual cycle.

This conversation is not just for girls, mind you. It is important for fathers to be able to speak to their children, girls or boys, about women's reproductive cycles in a knowledgeable and respectful manner. Seek support from female friends, groups, or counselors if necessary. We need to teach young boys about the female menstrual cycle—what it is and how to respect, nurture, and hold space for it—in positive and supportive ways. It is everyone's responsibility to make a positive change in perspective.

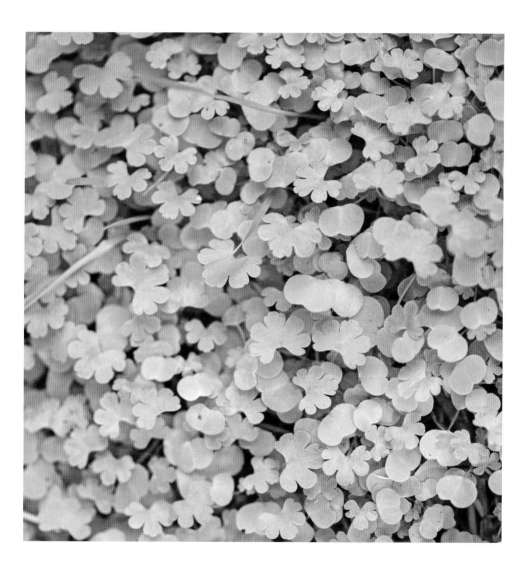

THE MENSTRUAL CYCLE

A female's hormone levels change every day. Although there is a steady pattern—estrogen rises for the first half of the cycle and falls during the second half—measurable levels are in fact different day to day. This is why true hormone testing needs to be performed over the duration of a month. You may truly feel like a different person every day, depending on what your hormones are doing!

The beginning of a new monthly cycle is the first day of your menses, the first day you bleed. It isn't when you notice a spot or two, but the first full bleeding day. Some bleed light, others bleed heavy, and there is a wide spectrum in between.

The first phase is the menstruation, or active bleeding phase. This phase coincides with the beginning of the next phase, the follicular phase. The follicular phase is when the ovaries produce a mature follicle to be released at ovulation. Ovulation is the release of that mature follicle, followed by the final, luteal, phase. The luteal phase is when the lining of the uterus thickens.

From a physiological perspective, if sperm does not fertilize the ovum (egg) that was released at ovulation, the egg simply decomposes and the menstrual cycle is initiated. The egg is released from the ovary and begins its slow and steady descent down through the fallopian tube to the uterus. Should the egg be fertilized, the luteal phase's buildup of the uterine lining will be utilized. The fertilized egg will attach itself somewhere in the uterine lining, and both the egg and the uterus will begin to release hormones to inhibit the menstrual cycle and allow the egg to grow.

When we consider the hormonal picture, it can be helpful to break the cycle down into a four-week picture. At the initiation, or first week, of the menstruation phase, estrogen levels are at ground zero. With estrogen (and progesterone) nonexistent, the pituitary gland is stimulated to release a hormone called follicular stimulating hormone (FSH). FSH is what triggers the ovary to begin maturing a new follicle into an ovum, which will eventually be released at ovulation. Within a couple of days of menstruation, estrogen begins to rise. Estrogen at this stage of the cycle often helps women feel relief from their menstruation complaints. Mood improves, optimism and energy increase, there's increased interest in being social or engaging in activities, and appetite is more manageable.

Estrogen continues to rise during the second week of the cycle as testosterone makes its appearance. Both have some truly beneficial side effects at this stage.

The continued rise in estrogen helps us think clearer and faster and continues to increase our desire to engage others socially. Estrogen at this point has been linked to a higher sense of self-assuredness and confidence. It is also a great time to go get those legs waxed, as estrogen can increase the release of certain endorphins that mask pain, making painful experiences much more bearable.

The increase in testosterone at this point leads to desire for intimate interactions, but it can also lead to a stronger sense of competitive or impulsive behaviors. None of these things need necessarily be viewed as negative. Testosterone can help us take a risk to achieve something we've wanted to accomplish, such as scuba diving for the first time or applying for a new job.

Ovulation typically occurs at the end of the second week. You might feel nothing, mild discomfort, or even a noticeable pain with the release of the egg.

At the beginning of the third week, we are now on the second half of the cycle. Unfortunately, this is typically the week things begin to go south for many women. Sometimes referred to as pre-PMS, many have mini versions of PMS symptoms. There may be a bit of irritation, a few random discouraging thoughts, and some food cravings here and there. Right before ovulation, estrogen surges and stimulates the pituitary gland to release a hormone called the luteinizing hormone (LH). LH triggers the egg to be released from the ovary. Estrogen drops a bit immediately following that surge, and this is what typically causes the pre-PMS symptoms. Thankfully, it doesn't take long, and estrogen begins to pick back up again to balance things out.

But the third week is also when progesterone begins to take center stage. It surpasses estrogen levels as it prepares the body for the possibility of a fertilized egg. The increase in progesterone can make you feel more tired, bloated, and perhaps not as sexually driven. On the flip side, increased progesterone helps many women feel mentally balanced and directed in their actions.

During the fourth week of the menstrual cycle, assuming there is no fertile egg implantation, both estrogen and progesterone begin to plummet. Not every woman feels premenstrual symptoms, but for those who do, the most common are fatigue, irritability, emotional sensitivity, depression, bloat, headaches, and cramps. Somewhere toward the end of four weeks, estrogen, progesterone, and testosterone are back to baseline 0, and the cycle begins again.

What is a normal menstrual cycle? And honestly, how can there be one answer to this question when we are so vastly different? There are some general guidelines for what falls into the normal range, but with genetics, culture, environmental choices, and exposures, it is virtually impossible to have a concrete answer.

Length of cycle: 26–35 days

Days of bleeding: 2–7

Menarche onset: Ages 10–14

The sooner you connect your emotional well-being with where you are in your menstrual cycle, the better. Forget the stereotyping of PMS and the comments, often made by men, such as "she must be on the rag," or "ignore her, she's on her period." Society has trained us to disconnect from our body and our ability to tap into what is really happening. Identifying how you feel throughout your cycle is worthwhile homework. When we are young, there is an enormous amount of processing occurring, and not just physically. It involves our physical, mental, and spiritual body as well as the world around us. If you can tap into how you process information emotionally—in particular, how you process it during the first half of your menstrual cycle compared to the latter half—you'll have valuable insight. Why? Because hormones can affect how we think, feel, and react to what is going on in our life.

Here's an example of hormones affecting how we act: When I was in my thirties, my mom came to live in the same city as I did, and I began to realize that whenever I was stressed out about something, I tended to dump on her a bit. Now, I love my mom dearly, but for some reason my hormonal stress response had decided my mom was an outlet for negative release. When I recognized the pattern, I knew my mom wasn't the problem at all; I was. I had to identify that how I handled stress was inappropriate, and that stress and hormones were driving my sense of frustration. Use a menstrual journal (see page 94) to help track your emotional patterns and your physical symptoms throughout your cycle to better identify your hormonal patterns and how they may be affecting you and others around you.

UNDERSTANDING UTERINE POSITIONING AND THE IMPORTANCE OF THE PELVIC FLOOR

Decades ago, the American Medical Association decided the uterus could be in one of four general positions in the abdominal cavity: anteverted, anteflexed, retroverted, or retroflexed. Anteverted means a uterus is midline and center, what I consider the true home of a uterus. Anteflexed is when the uterus is tipped forward, almost lying on the bladder. A retroverted uterus is slightly tipped backward, and a retroflexed uterus is bent backward. These terms are helpful, but ultimately your uterus should be midline and center in the pelvic bowl. So why are we finding them all over the place? The short answer is ligament problems, pregnancy, genetics, or trauma.

To illustrate this, I often sit in front of my patients and stretch my arms out and up a little to provide a visual. My body, I say, is the uterus. My arms are the fallopian tubes, and my hands are the ovaries. I then tip my body forward and show that if I am tipped forward, anteflexed, I am often sitting on top of the bladder. As my uterine lining increases during the month, I become heavier, which can lead to bladder irritation, frequency, or urgency. Then, I tip my body back and show that if I am tipped back, retroverted or retroflexed, I am pressing on the colon, nerves and muscles of the back, or the sacrum. This can lead to digestive disorders such as constipation and various types of pain, most commonly back pain. Any of these three positions can also cause potential implantation complications. In any of these positions, forward or back, the fallopian tubes may also be affected as they are stretched beyond their normal position.

And what if your uterus is tipped to one side or the other? I show this by tipping my body to the right or left. The arm (fallopian tube) on the opposite side I'm tipping to is really, really stretched. Meanwhile, the ovary on the side I'm tipped to is compressed by my body (the uterus). The tipped uterus can also be pinching the colon along the ascending or descending side. Any of these situations can potentially cause a host of menstrual or conception problems.

In Mayan abdominal therapy, Rosita Arvigo's work, it is believed that if a women's uterus is not midline and center, she herself is not centered. This therapy focuses on gently lifting the uterus to its correct midline position and strengthening the ligaments to support it. I have seen profound effects of this work, but none more so than the emotional release that comes with it.

Women often hold and store their life experiences and emotions in their uterus, and we have the gift of releasing them each month. With this release we can begin again both physically and emotionally. Honoring this tradition can be quite cathartic, especially when working through challenging times.

The treatment is an external abdominal massage that sometimes includes lower back massage as well. When I've performed this work with patients, the emotional release that often results is an honorable thing to bear witness to. Just thinking about it brings tears to my eyes. Women often report a strong sensation of energy, warmth, and circulation immediately afterwards, accompanied by many emotions or memories. Sensations they haven't felt in a long time, or perhaps ever, are acknowledged, and a deeper connection to themselves is initiated. If you are interested, visit the Arvigo Institute's website to find a local practitioner.

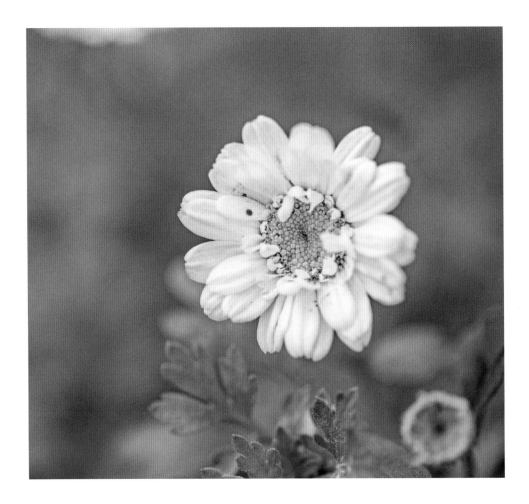

PELVIC FLOOR

The pelvic floor muscles support pelvic floor organs. These muscles assist in holding our bladder and bowel, contribute to sexual orgasm, stabilize all the surrounding connecting joints, pump in fresh blood and lymphatic tissue, and carry away metabolic waste. The health of this area is vital to the reproductive, urinary, and lower intestinal systems. If there is weakness or stagnation, various problems can arise. When tension is present, oxygen and blood supply can be diminished.

A modality that focuses on connection and the release of stored experiences and emotions in this area is the holistic pelvic care originated by Tami Kent. Her in-depth book *Wild Feminine* is a great tool for anyone interested in the concept of release through deeper connection with our bodies. In Tami's philosophy, pelvic floor work restores balance in the female pelvis to increase the strength of core muscles, enhance pelvic energetic vitality, improve sensation, provide support for infertility, recover from pregnancy and childbirth, and reconnect to the beauty of the pelvic bowl. This therapy is focused on relaxing built up tension in the pelvic floor and uterine muscles. When we tense any muscle for a prolonged period, it begins to create a holding of the muscle in that tense way. By inserting one or two fingers into the vaginal canal and applying gentle pressure to tense areas, we help the muscle begin to relax. This allows new blood flow and oxygen to the area, increasing relaxation.

Working through past abuse or trauma can be frightening, overwhelming, and even at times too much to handle. Utilizing any of the positive female practices mentioned in chapter 1, Mayan abdominal massage, or Tami Kent's pelvic floor work can aid the process. Practitioners who work within the realm of uterine health are often in tune with emotions that come up when talking about a woman's reproductive health, much less in touching any part of her body. When we experience trauma, even on the smallest scale, verbally, physically, or mentally, it often gets trapped in our body. We take in the experience and seal it off so that it won't damage us further. Whether that works for you or not, the experience is trapped on the physical level. This can lead to a multitude of negative effects, such as pain, dysfunction, repeated emotional responses, and, at the extreme, the inability to move forward in certain areas of life. Even if the trauma occurred years ago, symptoms can arise down the road. Another therapy that I'm a huge fan of, which might help, is Rosen therapy.

When I was twenty-five I moved from the Midwest to Seattle. I knew not a soul in Seattle and was thrilled about it. When I was young, I loved the opportunity to leave a place, take all that I had learned, shed the no-longer-needed aspects of myself, and start over. The universe was guiding my entire Seattle experience, and one night I ended up at a party. I wasn't the best at small talk, and thankfully there was music to fill the void. But I did end up speaking to a young woman about healing paths, and she told me about Rosen therapy. Taking the signal from the universe, I found a Rosen therapist and scheduled an appointment.

Rosen therapy is a type of bodywork that is distinguished by its gentle, direct touch. You are fully clothed and simply rest on a massage table. Using his or her hands, the practitioner focuses on finding chronic muscle tension in the body. Practitioners gently touch and feel the muscles, and when they find tension they "hold" the muscle. There really isn't a better way to describe it. This "holding" goes on for as long as it takes for relaxation to occur and the breath to deepen. Unconscious feelings, attitudes, and memories can come up. At first, it can be a bit disarming, as what comes up isn't always obvious trauma that you are working through. As the treatment continues, habitual tension and old patterns may be released, leading to a cathartic feeling of release, ease, and understanding.

When I arrived, the practitioner explained the process a bit and then asked me to lay on the table. Then the work began. She subtly moved her hands to different muscles on my body and just sort of held them. First my neck muscles, then my shoulders, and then my calves. With each group, there was an overwhelming amount of release, not just physically but emotionally as well. I had no idea what was happening, but it felt safe and good. The practitioner spoke to me gently throughout the session and encouraged me to speak when things came up, but I was nowhere near ready for such vulnerability. I left feeling like a completely different person. The biggest impact was the realization that we hold *a lot* of stuff in our body instead of processing it through and out. Without releasing it, how can we ever be truly healthy?

LEAVING BEHIND OBC: A STORY

In my early twenties, I decided I no longer wished to be on birth control pills. I'd felt for a while that I was taking something that wasn't allowing my body to follow its natural rhythm. I didn't have any issues while taking oral birth control; I had short cycles, no cramping, and the protection from pregnancy. But I couldn't ignore this growing sensation that my body didn't really want to be taking the drug. Thus began my journey of stopping the pill and trying to get my menstrual cycle back. For four years I had no menses. Four years. At the time, no one had an answer for me. I went to three different doctors; all told me: "You are young, you are healthy, it's normal, don't worry about it, and it'll work itself out." I was frustrated. It didn't feel normal. I didn't feel healthy, and I had the gnawing sensation that it wasn't going to "work itself out."

The fourth doctor did an ultrasound and revealed that my ovaries looked like waffles. Or at least that is what they looked like to me. I was told that I had polycystic ovary syndrome, PCOS. Treatment? I was told there was nothing I could do, but not to worry. When I wanted to get pregnant, just come back and he'd give me something to stimulate ovulation.

Once again, I left a doctor's office frustrated. It was time to take matters into my own hands. When I began to research PCOS, I realized I only had one defining symptom: no menstrual cycle. And so I started off on my road to natural medicine. I read everything I could about herbs, acupuncture, essential oils, massage, and old nature cures. I decided to go with acupuncture because it resonated with me, and because in the Midwest in the 1990s, I didn't have access to anything else. Fortunately, there was one acupuncturist in my state; I only had to drive one hour each way to see him, so acupuncture it was.

As it turned out, you had to be a licensed MD to practice acupuncture in Nebraska at the time, and my acupuncturist practiced at the medical school. A very nice man entered the room, and I quickly noticed his relaxed state. He wasn't in a hurry. He actually looked me in the eye and listened intently when I spoke. He then guided me through the treatment, always telling me what was going to happen before it happened. And as crazy as it seemed, I laid there while the nice man put needles into my body. I was scared, excited, and nervous. But after about ten minutes, I was completely asleep. I woke up forty-five minutes later and drove home. Two days later, I had my first menstrual cycle in four years.

Although my first acupuncture session obviously had a huge impact on me, not all natural modalities, including herbs, will be life altering. I have dedicated my life to herbs because, in my experience, they are effective, and I have seen it time and time again.

Every woman's journey with her body and menstrual cycle is an insightful story, even when there is pain. I love to encourage my patients to create a menstrual journal. Whether you are as regular as clockwork or attempting to balance out your cycles, this journal is a wonderful tool. Some women simply record the basics, such as when they start and stop bleeding, what days they experience certain symptoms, and when ovulation occurs. Others include moon cycles, memories and special events, photos, sketches, and/or poems. Your day-to-day feelings are of great value to reflect upon. After a few months, you may identify patterns within your cycle, associating certain emotions with certain points of the cycle. You can download all sorts of apps for your phone these days, if that makes it easier. Personally, I prefer the look and feel of something tangible. My journal is a deeper reflection of myself—what is going on in my life, as well as my attempt to stay grounded and connected to my body.

In this chapter, I'll provide many recipes for young girls and women to support the menstrual cycle and decrease the common complaints that may arise during this phase of life. Keep in mind that hormones take time to shift into a new pattern. Consistent herbal treatment for three to six months is sometimes necessary. Don't expect a quick fix in this department.

Common Physical Complaints of the Dawning Phase

Trouble regulating cycles	Headaches
Painful menstruation	Mood swings
Spotting between periods	Bacterial infections
Breast tenderness	Yeast infections
Bloating	Need for birth control
Need for hormone tonics	

REGULATING MENSES

Once menstruation begins, it can come like clockwork each month or it can come and go, skipping months or stopping from time to time. Sometimes it takes a while before the new way of doing something regulates. The body is no exception, and there is no need for alarm if it takes up to a year for a new menstrual cycle to become regular. If at the one-year mark there are still inconsistencies in flow, length, or duration of the cycle, it is worth seeing your practitioner for supportive treatment. Here are a few options to encourage hormonal balance and regular cycles.

Stock your home herbal pantry with the following for regulating menses:

Angelica root

Bupleurum root

Burdock root

Chamomile flowers

Cinnamon bark

Dong Quai root

Lemongrass

Motherwort

Nettle leaf

Partridgeberry

Peppermint

Rosehips

Vitex berry

Yellow Dock root

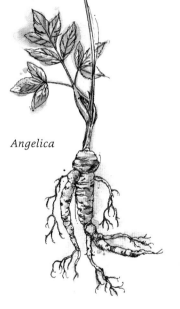

Angelica

Where to Begin: A Simple Protocol for Menstrual Regulation

If you know your cycle somewhat, drink Peppermint tea days 1 to 15 and Chamomile tea day 16 to the first day of bleeding. These two herbs support both the first and second halves of the menstrual cycle and are sometimes all the body needs.

The uterus is a larger grouping of smooth muscle. It contracts during menstruation and labor and stretches as an increase in uterine lining occurs each month during pregnancy. Magnesium targets smooth muscle and can calm down intense contractions. Because cell salts are sublingual, meaning they quickly pass through the sublingual tissues under the tongue, they immediately enter the bloodstream and go to whatever area is needed. This allows them to reach their target destination and begin to reduce contractions extremely quickly.

I cannot tell you how many patients and customers I've recommended magnesium cell salts to for uterine cramping, with incredible results. So many grateful women have returned saying it is the first time they have had a positive result so quickly.

The recommended dosage is 6 pellets under the tongue every 20 minutes until cramping subsides.

MENSTRUAL REGULATOR TEA

Drink this tea daily to work on your estrogen/progesterone balance, which will create regularity in your monthly cycle.

1 ounce (28 g) dried vitex berries	YIELD: 4 ounces (112 g)
½ ounce (14 g) dried motherwort	Place all ingredients except the honey
¼ ounce (7 g) dried dong quai	in an airtight glass jar; store at room temperature.
1 ounce (28 g) dried rosehips	perature. Make medicinal strength (see
1 ounce (28 g) dried lemongrass	page 245) and sweeten to taste with
Honey to taste	honey; drink 2 or 3 cups each day for
	12 weeks.

LIVER SUPPORT FOR MONTHLY FLOW TINCTURE

If you notice fluctuations in flow amount or the number of days in your cycles, your liver may need to be supported as well.

1 tablespoon (15 ml) vitex berry tincture	YIELD: 1 ounce (28 ml)
1 teaspoon (5 ml) angelica root tincture	Combine all ingredients together in a
1 teaspoon (5 ml) yellow dock root tincture	1-ounce (28 ml) amber dropper bottle;
1 teaspoon (5 ml) bupleurum root tincture	gently shake to mix. Take 1 dropperful
	3 times per day for 3 to 6 months.

Castor Oil Packs

Castor oil packs are a wonderful treatment for all menstrual complaints. They bind excess estrogen, stimulate the immune system, and help reduce prostaglandin hormones (increased in those who have painful cramps). See page 102 for more.

LITTLE TO LOW BLOOD FLOW TINCTURE

When your cycle produces little to no blood, you may run the risk of not eliminating each month's accumulation of uterine lining. This means 1 day or less of bleeding, or only spotting throughout your menses. Having 2 to 4 days of mild to moderate flow is considered normal and is a great sign that your body is reserving its essences without excessive blood flow. But when your flow is less than that, you may wish to boost blood nutrients and hormone patterns to encourage healthy release.

1½ teaspoons (7 ml) yellow dock root tincture

1 teaspoon (5 ml) dong quai root tincture

1 teaspoon (5 ml) nettle leaf tincture

1 teaspoon (5 ml) partridgeberry tincture

1 teaspoon (5 ml) burdock root tincture

½ teaspoon (3 ml) cinnamon tincture

YIELD: 2 ounces (60 ml)

Combine all ingredients in a 2-ounce (60 ml) amber tincture bottle. Take 1 dropperful 3 times per day.

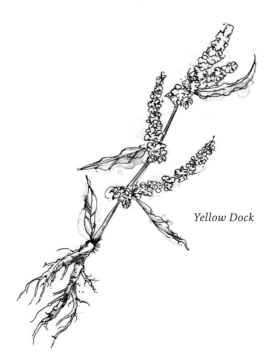

Yellow Dock

PAINFUL MENSTRUATION

Having the tools to combat menstrual pain, whether mild or severe, can be life changing. Pain can be caused by hormone imbalance, increased prostaglandins, uterine position, endometriosis, fibroids, cysts, emotional trauma, past surgeries, and on and on. I've had my fair share of patients with debilitating menstrual pain, and I work hard to try to help them identify the herbs that can support them. Sometimes, energetic medicines such as flower essences or craniosacral therapy is necessary; other times, mental therapy or physical therapies such as pelvic floor work are the keys to identifying the causes. I encourage you to do whatever it takes within reason to find the support your body needs. Pain is a clear sign that your body is asking for help.

Stock your home herbal pantry with the following for painful menstruation:

Black Cohosh	Hops strobiles	Silk Tassel
Burdock root	Licorice	Valerian root
California Poppy	Milk Thistle	White Oak bark
Crampbark	Partridgeberry	Wild Yam

Where to Begin: A Simple Protocol for Menstrual Pain

Cell salts are a whole different topic from herbal medicine, but it's one worth mentioning when it comes to menstrual pain. Cell salts are minute dosages of the exact trace minerals that are naturally found in our bodies. The theory is that when we are deficient in these trace minerals, organ functions can degrade and symptoms arise out of their dysfunction. There are twelve cell salts available for purchase, and I'm sure you are familiar with at least three: calcium, magnesium, and phosphorus.

The uterus is a larger grouping of smooth muscle. It contracts during menstruation and labor and stretches as an increase in uterine lining occurs each month during pregnancy. Magnesium targets smooth muscle and can calm down intense contractions. Because cell salts are sublingual, meaning they quickly pass through the sublingual tissues under the tongue, they immediately enter the bloodstream and go to whatever area is needed. This allows them to reach their target destination and begin to reduce contractions extremely quickly.

I cannot tell you how many patients and customers I've recommended magnesium cell salts to for uterine cramping, with incredible results. So many grateful women have returned saying it is the first time they have had a positive result so quickly.

The recommended dosage is 6 pellets under the tongue every 20 minutes until cramping subsides.

CRAMPING RELIEF TINCTURE

Herbal tinctures are another option for quick relief. They bypass the digestive system and go to work quickly, especially for acute pain. For acute situations, use this tincture for temporary relief of menstrual cramping.

1½ teaspoons (8 ml) crampbark tincture	YIELD: 1 ounce (28 ml)
1½ teaspoons (8 ml) silk tassel tincture	Combine all ingredients in a 1-ounce (28 ml)
1 teaspoon (5 ml) black cohosh tincture	amber dropper bottle. Take 1 to 2 dropperfuls
1 teaspoon (5 ml) white oak bark tincture	as needed, not to exceed 6 doses per day.
¾ teaspoon (4 ml) California poppy tincture	

CRAMPING TONIC FORMULA

Estrogen excess is often the culprit when it comes to cramping. This formula is targeted to reduce estrogen, and it's intended to be taken all month long.

2 teaspoons (10 ml) partridgeberry tincture	YIELD: 2 ounces (60 ml)
1 teaspoon (5 ml) burdock root tincture	Combine all ingredients in a 2-ounce (60 ml)
1 teaspoon (5 ml) wild yam tincture	amber dropper bottle. Take 1 dropperful
1 teaspoon (5 ml) milk thistle tincture	3 times per day.
1 teaspoon (5 ml) licorice tincture	

TOPICAL CRAMPING RELIEF OIL

Use this formula to provide soothing relief from menstrual cramping pain.

1 ounce (28 g) dried crampbark	YIELD: 1 to 2 cups (235 to 475 ml)
1 ounce (28 g) dried valerian root	Preheat oven to 170°F (77°C). Place herbs in
¼ ounce (7 g) dried hops strobiles	a glass baking dish and pour enough olive oil
1 to 2 cups (235 to 475 ml) olive oil	over them to cover by 1 to 2 inches (3 to 5 cm).
15 drops chamomile essential oil	Bake for 4 hours. Allow to cool and then strain
10 drops ylang-ylang essential oil	into a storage container. Add essential oils and
5 drops rose essential oil	stir well. Use 1 to 4 tablespoons (15 to 60 ml)
	of oil when needed to relieve cramping pain.

SPOTTING BETWEEN PERIODS

Spotting can be caused by hormonal imbalance, thyroid issues, ovarian problems, fibroids, or more serious pathologies. If you haven't reached menopause and there is no accompanying pain, pregnancy, fever, or increasing frequency, spotting is most likely a normal abnormality. Birth control methods often cause spotting as hormone levels fluctuate.

Stock your home herbal pantry with the following for menstrual spotting:

Chamomile flowers	Red Raspberry	Spearmint leaf
Lady's Mantle leaf	Shatavari root	Vitex berry
Peppermint	Shepherd's Purse	

TONIC TEA FOR OCCASIONAL SPOTTING

Spotting throughout the month needs to be addressed by supporting the hormones of the reproductive cycle. Drink this tea daily to find hormonal balance. Keep in mind that shifting hormones don't happen overnight. Be patient and consistent with treatments.

1 ounce (28 g) dried vitex berries

1 ounce (28 g) dried red raspberry

½ ounce (14 g) dried lady's mantle leaf

½ ounce (14 g) dried shatavari root

1 ounce (28 g) dried spearmint

1 ounce (28 g) dried peppermint

YIELD: 5 ounces (140 g)

Stir all ingredients together; store in a glass jar. Make medicinal strength (see page 245) and drink 2 cups daily for 8 to 12 weeks.

SPOTTING STOPPER TINCTURE

When spotting comes and goes throughout the menstrual cycle, it is often a sign of hormone imbalance. Use this formula to astringe the uterus to stop bleeding when it is not regular menses time.

1 teaspoon (15 ml) shepherd's purse tincture

2 teaspoons (10 ml) chamomile flower tincture

1 teaspoon (5 ml) red raspberry leaf tincture

YIELD: 1 once (28 ml)

Mix all ingredients together in a 1-ounce (28 ml) amber dropper bottle. Take 1 to 2 dropperfuls every 20 minutes until bleeding subsides. Most women experience a slowing or stopping of bleeding after 2 to 4 doses. Do not exceed 8 doses.

BREAST TENDERNESS

As with any cyclic symptom, it is best to treat breast tenderness before it arises. Tenderness can come at any point during the menstrual cycle, but it is most prevalent during the week leading up to bleeding.

Stock your home herbal pantry with the following for breast tenderness:

Boswellia

Cleavers leaf

Dandelion leaf

Lemon Balm leaf

Nettle leaf

Turmeric root

BREAST COMFORT CAPSULES

These capsules can be used throughout the month or the week preceding menstruation to decrease symptoms of pain, swelling, and tenderness.

½ ounce (14 g) turmeric root powder	**YIELD:** 200 capsules
½ ounce (14 g) boswellia powder	Stir all ingredients in a bowl; fill empty
¼ ounce (7 g) dandelion leaf powder	vegetable capsules with the mixture.
¼ ounce (7 g) cleavers leaf powder	Take 3 capsules, 3 times per day.

SOOTHING TEA

Drink this simple blend as needed for temporary relief in breast swelling.

1 ounce (28 g) dried nettle leaf	**YIELD:** 4 ounces (112 g)
1 ounce (28 g) dried dandelion leaf	Combine all herbs together; store in a glass
½ ounce (14 g) dried cleavers leaf	jar. Make by the cup: Steep 2 teaspoons
1½ ounces (42 g) dried lemon balm	(3 g) in 12 ounces (355 ml) of boiling water, covered, for 10 minutes.

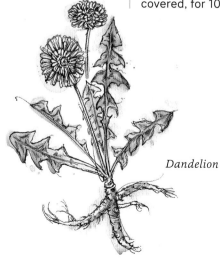

Dandelion

BLOATING

Bloating is the sensation of abdominal swelling or the feeling of being unusually full even if you haven't eaten. Bloating typically isn't painful, but it is uncomfortable. Fluctuations in hormones are often to blame. As we move through the month and estrogen and progesterone rise and fall, water can accumulate, leading to clothes not fitting and a feeling of heaviness throughout the body. Whenever bloating is present, we need to consider our diet, as certain foods lead to abdominal inflammation and bloating. Take note to see if your bloating consistently occurs after eating. Wheat and dairy are common culprits, but even vegetables and proteins can cause bloating. Using herbs to balance the hormones (see "Hormone Tonics") is your best approach to combating bloat, but also consider the following recipes to help make you more comfortable.

Stock your home herbal pantry with the following for menstrual bloating:

Calamus root	Dandelion leaf	Fennel seed
Caraway seed	Dandelion root	Peppermint leaf

BLOAT RELIEF TEA

Have a cuppa to relieve yourself of the uncomfortable abdominal fullness often felt during premenstrual times.

1 ounce (28 g) dried dandelion leaf	YIELD: 4 ounces (112 g)
1 ounce (28 g) dried calamus root	Stir all herbs together; store in a glass jar. Make by the cup as needed: Steep 2 teaspoons (3 g) in 12 ounces (355 ml) of boiling water, covered, for 10 minutes.
½ ounce (14 g) dried dandelion root	
½ ounce (14 g) dried fennel seed	
1 ounce (28 g) dried peppermint	

CASTOR OIL PACK FOR BLOATING

This is a warm and healing treatment targeted for longer-lasting bloat relief.

1 ounce (28 g) dried fennel seed	YIELD: 1 to 2 cups (235 to 475 ml)
½ ounce (14 g) dried caraway seed	Preheat oven to 170°F (77°C). Place herbs in a glass baking dish; pour enough castor oil over them to cover by 1 to 2 inches (3 to 5 cm). Bake for 4 hours. Allow to cool and then strain into a storage container. Add 10 drops of ginger essential oil. Apply nightly or as needed for 30 to 45 minutes.
½ ounce (14 g) dried calamus root	
2 cups (475 ml) castor oil	
10 drops ginger essential oil	

QUICK RELIEF BLOATING TINCTURE

Feeling the abdominal squeeze? This formula is blended for quick temporary relief of bloating.

1 tablespoon (15 ml) chamomile flowers tincture

1 teaspoon (5 ml) turmeric root tincture

1 teaspoon (5 ml) dandelion leaf tincture

½ teaspoon (2.5 ml) ginger root tincture

½ teaspoon (2.5 ml) anise seed tincture

YIELD: 1 ounce (28 ml)
Combine all ingredients in a 1-ounce (28 ml) amber dropper bottle. Take 1 dropperful 3 times per day or as needed.

HORMONE TONICS

Sometimes, women's cycles veer off track ever so slightly for unknown reasons. Throughout my 20s, for example, my menstrual cycle would switch from starting on the full moon to the new moon each fall. Nothing out of the ordinary would trigger this change, but I began to support my hormone body each fall. I used hormone tonics to nourish and tone the reproductive, endocrine, and liver systems as reverence for my body. It's easy to forget about how much our body does for us every day. Taking time to acknowledge and care for it even when nothing is wrong, per se, is the key to preventive health.

Stock your home herbal pantry with the following for hormone tonics:

Barberry

Blue Vervain leaf

Chamomile flowers

Cinnamon bark

Ginger root

Hawthorn berry

Lemon Balm leaf

Maca

Oat Straw

Partridgeberry

Tribulus

Vitex berry

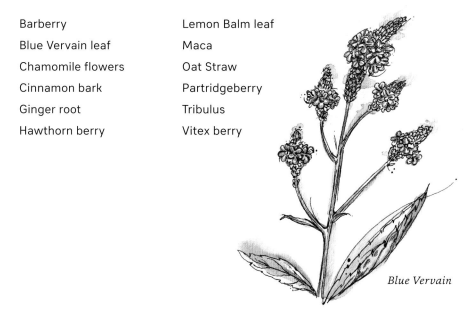

Blue Vervain

FEMALE TONIC TEA

Drink this tea daily to support the reproductive and nervine systems.

2 ounces (56 g) dried blue vervain leaf	YIELD: 4 ounces (112 g)
½ ounce (14 g) dried chamomile flowers	Combine all ingredients; store in a glass jar.
½ ounce (14 g) dried lemon balm leaf	Make medicinal strength (see page 245)
½ ounce (14 g) dried oat straw	and drink 2 cups daily for 3 to 4 weeks, 1 to
½ ounce (14 g) dried vitex berry	3 times per year.

FEMALE TONIC TINCTURE

Feeling a little off in your cycle? Maybe your cycle has shortened or lengthened? Maybe stress is higher than normal and you're wondering if your estrogen is a bit high? These are all good times to take this blend, which offers balance and support to the liver and the reproductive system.

2 teaspoons (10 ml) partridgeberry tincture	YIELD: 1 ounce (28 ml)
2 teaspoons (10 ml) tribulus tincture	Combine all ingredients in a 1-ounce (28 ml)
1 teaspoon (5 ml) barberry tincture	amber dropper bottle. Take 1 dropperful
1 teaspoon (5 ml) hawthorn berry tincture	3 times per day for 4 to 6 weeks as needed.

MACA LATTE FOR HORMONAL BALANCE

Maca is known for its endocrine balancing effects, and this is a great way to take it. Whether you have obvious signs of hormonal imbalance, such as PMS, cramping, or acne, or you just want to do the endocrine system good, maca makes a great daily tonic. Smooth and creamy, it's a great cup to start the day. Caution: It's very addicting!

1 cup (235 ml) any milk (My favorites are hemp or almond milk.)	YIELD: 1 serving
5 teaspoons (9 g) maca powder	Combine all ingredients except coconut oil in a mixing bowl. Whisk by hand or blend
1 teaspoon fresh ginger, sliced	with a blender or an immersion blender.
1 teaspoon ground cinnamon	Transfer mixture to a saucepan; heat uncov-
2 pitted dates (Medjool dates are a good choice.)	ered, stirring frequently, over low heat.
½ teaspoon (2.5 ml) vanilla extract	Add coconut oil and stir until melted.
1 tablespoon (14 g) coconut oil	

HEADACHES

As someone who had chronic headaches growing up, I can relate if you are a fellow sufferer. Looking back on it, food and hormones most likely caused my daily headaches. I had no other resources, so ibuprofen was part of my daily life. There are many reasons that headaches come on, but for this chapter, we'll focus on three: hormone imbalance, liver insufficiency, and the Chinese medicine theory of blood deficiency.

Hormonal imbalances such as increased estrogen, lowered progesterone, decreased cortisol, and thyroid problems can all cause headaches. Naturally, balancing out and supporting the endocrine system will help decrease headache frequency. Although prostaglandins aren't classified as hormones per se, if they are present in excess amounts they can also lead to headaches due to their ability to constrict blood vessels and increase sensitivity to pain.

Liver insufficiency is caused when there is an accumulation of metabolic waste, hormones, and/or chemical precursors due to lack of efficiency in clearing them through the liver detoxification pathways. Because these things are usually processed and utilized or released through elimination, they end up causing trouble when they remain in the body. Helping the liver process more efficiently is necessary. Herbs can help, but remember: Sleep is vital for the liver to do its work!

In Chinese medicine, blood deficiency is defined as a pattern in which the yin aspects of the blood are lacking. When this occurs, the yang aspects of the body take over, often leading to headaches. If you experience dizziness, headaches, scanty menstruation, pale complexion, and sleep issues, consider seeking out your local acupuncturist for treatment.

See "Hormone Tonics," regulating hormone, and liver support recipes for more options to help with headaches.

Stock your home herbal pantry with the following for hormonal headaches:

Black Cohosh root	Lobelia leaf	Valerian root
Blessed Thistle leaf	Oat Straw	Vitex berry
Hop Strobiles	Peppermint leaf	White Willow bark
Lavender flower	Turmeric root	

ACUTE HEADACHE HERBAL TINCTURE

Use this tincture for temporary relief from headache pain.

1 tablespoon (15 ml) white willow bark tincture	YIELD: 1 once (28 ml)
1 teaspoon (5 ml) lavender flower tincture	Combine all ingredients in a 1-ounce (28 ml)
1 teaspoon (5 ml) peppermint tincture	amber dropper bottle. Take 1 dropperful
1 teaspoon (5 ml) hops tincture	every 30 minutes until headache subsides. Do not exceed 6 doses per day.

HORMONAL HEADACHE TONIC TINCTURE

Menstrual headaches tend to come on right before, during, or at the finish of bleeding. Because research shows that hormone fluctuations are typically the cause of these types of headaches, using this formula throughout the month gives it the best chance to balance those hormones, resulting in a decrease of headaches or a decrease in pain with headaches.

1½ teaspoons (8 ml) blessed thistle leaf tincture	YIELD: 1 ounce (28 ml)
1½ teaspoons (8 ml) black cohosh root tincture	Combine all ingredients in a 1-ounce (28 ml)
1½ teaspoons (8 ml) turmeric root tincture	amber dropper bottle. Take 1 dropperful
½ teaspoon (3 ml) oat straw tincture	3 times per day.
½ teaspoon (3 ml) vitex berry tincture	

HEADACHE BALM

Rub a bit of this onto the temples and nape of the neck for relief from headache pain and pressure.

1 ounce (28 g) dried black cohosh	YIELD: 8 ounces (224 g)
1 ounce (28 g) dried valerian	Preheat oven to 170°F (77°C). Place herbs in
¼ ounce (7 g) dried hops	a glass baking dish; pour enough olive oil over
¼ ounce (7 g) dried lobelia	them to cover by 1 to 2 inches (3 to 5 cm).
1½ cups (355 ml) olive oil	Bake at 170°F (77°C) for 4 hours. Allow to
1 to 1½ ounces (28 to 42 g) beeswax	cool and then strain into a saucepan. Heat
1 ounce (28 ml) poplar oil	uncovered over low heat. Add beeswax,
20 to 40 drops rosemary essential oil, to scent preference	stirring until completely melted. Add poplar and rosemary essential oils; pour into a storage container.

MOOD SWINGS

There is no doubt that our personal lives greatly affect both the mood we project out into the world and our sense of well-being. When we live satisfied lives, our abilities to communicate, engage, and manifest come from a grounded and centered place. When we are in an unhappy job or relationship or our standard of living is compromised, it becomes increasingly harder to find balance within the world and ourselves. Combine this with a hormonal imbalance and we can feel downright out of place all the time. Feelings such as insecurity, anger, sadness, and hopelessness can pervade our daily existence and can make day-to-day living a struggle. One of the best things you can do to help is learning to identify when your hormones are acting out of balance. It is hard enough connecting to our true selves as we grow up without having to navigate hormonal imbalances. Be keen to observe yourself if extreme swings are occurring. When do they occur? Is there a pattern in relationship to your menstrual cycle? What is happening in your personal life to exaggerate your feelings?

Stock your home herbal pantry with the following for mood swings:

Chamomile flowers	Lemongrass	St. John's Wort
Ginkgo leaf	Passionflower leaf	Vitex berry
Lavender flower	Schizandra berry	Wood Betony
Lemon Balm	Skullcap leaf	

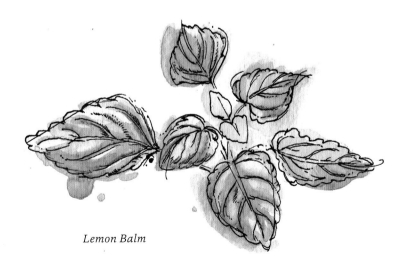

Lemon Balm

MAY THE LONG TIME SUN SHINE UPON YOU TEA

In kundalini meditation, there is a song that you typically end each class with. As you close your practice, the song reminds you that you are a radiant being with a lot to offer yourself and those around you. When we aren't feeling our best, try this tea and remind yourself of all the best parts of who you are.

1 ounce (28 g) dried passionflower

1 ounce (28 g) dried ginkgo leaf

½ ounce (14 g) dried St. John's wort

1 ounce (28 g) dried lemongrass

½ ounce (14 g) dried chamomile

¼ ounce (7 g) dried lavender flower

YIELD: 4 ounces (112 g)

Combine all herbs together; store in a glass jar. Make tea by the cup as needed: Steep 2 teaspoons (3 g) of tea in 12 ounces (355 ml) boiling water, covered, for 10 minutes.

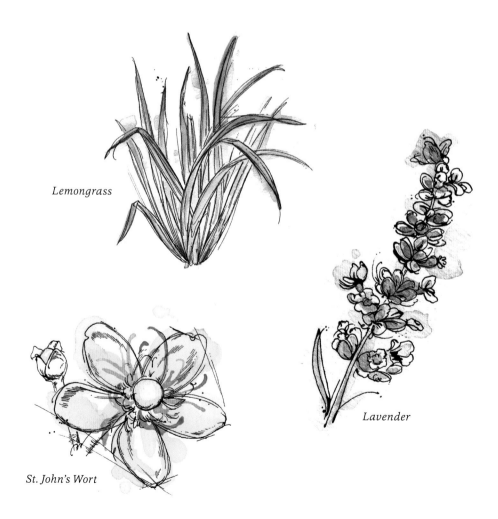

Lemongrass

Lavender

St. John's Wort

HERBAL MOOD TONIC

When stabilizing your mood is a real struggle, you can try this formula, which supports the nervous system and adrenal glands. It's not to be taken with selective serotonin reuptake inhibitors (SSRIs). Consult your practitioner if you believe you may be clinically depressed.

2½ teaspoons (12 ml) St. John's wort tincture	YIELD: 1 ounce (28 ml)
1 teaspoon (5 ml) lemon balm tincture	Blend all ingredients in a 1-ounce (28 ml)
1 teaspoon (5 ml) wood betony tincture	amber dropper bottle. Take 1 dropperful
1 teaspoon (5 ml) skullcap tincture	3 times per day.
1 teaspoon (5 ml) schizandra berry tincture	
½ teaspoon (3 ml) vitex berry tincture	

PLEASANT MOOD ESSENTIAL OIL BLEND

Citrus essential oils have been known to uplift the mood for decades. Try placing a drop or two of this blend into your palms, rubbing them together, and taking two or three deep inhalations. When we smell essential oils, our scent center, or olfactory, in our nose gets stimulated and sends messages up to the brain to react in certain ways.

½ teaspoon (3 ml) bergamot oil	YIELD: 2 teaspoons (10 ml)
½ teaspoon (3 ml) sweet orange oil	Combine all oils into an essential oil bottle.
½ teaspoon (3 ml) clary sage oil	Use as described above or in a diffuser,
¼ teaspoon (1 ml) frankincense oil	as desired.
¼ teaspoon (1 ml) lavender oil	

Flower Essences

When our emotions are getting the best of us, it is time for self-reflection. One of my favorite set of tools to help work through tough emotional terrains are flower essences. Flower essences work to help process through emotions that we haven't quite been able to get a grasp on. Being able to identify one emotion is all you need to begin. The Flower Essence Society is an incredible resource for more information.

VAGINAL HEALTH

Our vaginas are as close to personal as personal can get. Depending on culture, religion, upbringing, and our opportunity for self-expression, our vaginas closely reflect deeper truths about ourselves. Just saying the word *vagina* can make some people uncomfortable. It is a body part that has often been stigmatized into negative realms. And women are the key to changing that stigma. It doesn't mean we need to wear vagina T-shirts wherever we go (though if you want to, go for it!), but it does mean we should use the word when we are talking about, well, vaginas. Let's all get comfy with it, shall we?

There are several repeat offenders that occur within the vaginal track and cause imbalance. A big player is pH, as it can quickly throw off vaginal flora, leading to either bacterial or yeast infections. Considering diet, clothing, stress, and hygiene habits are important, but sometimes herbs are just the support a woman needs.

VAGINAL STEAM

While this practice is not exclusive to Mayan culture, it is there I learned of it. A vaginal steam is a wonderful treatment not only for the vagina but also for the womb and for the woman. It is best done in meditation, giving yourself full permission to relax and embrace yourself. It's helpful any time, particularly pre- and post-menstrual cycle. And it's a thoughtful gift to give a friend—offer to orchestrate this delicate and respectful treatment so she can feel fully cared for. There are variations on this blend of herbs; feel free to research and adapt. You will need a slatted chair or a vaginal steam chair, which is a chair with a hole in the center. Basically, you need a chair that will allow the steam to come through it.

Ingredients	Instructions
1 ounce (28 g) dried rosemary leaf 1 ounce (28 g) dried holy basil 1 ounce (28 g) dried calendula 1 ounce (28 g) dried rose petals	YIELD: 1 vaginal steam treatment Bring a large stockpot of water almost to a boil; turn off the heat and add herbs. Give the mixture a quick stir and close the lid. Let steep for 15 minutes. Make yourself a cup of tea. Move the pot beneath the chair you'll be sitting on, in a quiet, private place. You will need to be undressed from the waist down. Get yourself comfortable and situated on your chair. Wrap a heavy blanket around

(continued)

you, ensuring that it falls to the ground to encase the steam, not allowing it to go anywhere but up. Place a footstool or pillow or two in front of you. Once you are ready, remove the lid from the pot and rest your feet up on your pillows. Relax. Breathe. Sip your tea. Allow the steam to circulate its way to your bum and vagina. I tend to encourage a rest of 30 to 45 minutes, but you can decide how long to stay.

VAGINAL FISSURE SALVE

At times, tiny tears called fissures can occur after sex. Although tiny, they can burn and hurt significantly. Using this salve can heal them quickly and provide the cool-down needed during repair. I personally prefer not to add essential oils to this formula, but if I were going to, I would add either rose or chamomile for their gentle healing support.

¼ ounce (7 g) dried calendula

¼ ounce (7 g) dried lavender

¼ ounce (7 g) dried chickweed

¼ ounce (7 g) dried rose petals

1 cup (235 ml) olive oil

1 ounce (28 g) beeswax

YIELD: 8 ounces (235 ml)

Preheat oven to 170°F (77°C). Place herbs in a shallow glass baking dish and pour olive oil over them. Bake for 4 hours. Strain and transfer to a saucepan. Add beeswax over low heat and stir until melted. Transfer to a lidded storage container; let cool completely before closing. Apply a spot of salve to the irritated or inflamed area, 1 to 3 times per day until healed.

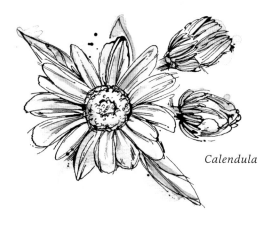

Calendula

VAGINAL INFECTIONS

Because bacterial vaginosis and yeast infections tend to occur most often in our 20s and 30s, they are included here, but also refer to the "Support" chapter for additional recipes.

Stock your home herbal pantry with the following for vaginal infections:

Boric acid (not borax)	Lavender flowers	Rose petals
Calendula flowers	Marshmallow root	Slippery Elm bark
Chickweed	Myrrh	Turmeric root
Comfrey leaf	Pau d'Arco	Usnea lichen
Echinacea root	Peppermint leaf	Yarrow flowers
Goldenseal root	Plantain leaf	

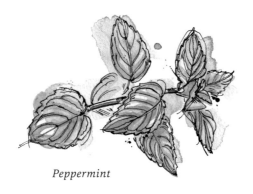

Peppermint

BACTERIAL INFECTIONS

Bacterial infections, affectionately known as BV, include such symptoms as an abnormal amount of vaginal discharge, the discharge being thin and grayish white, vaginal odor, irritation of vaginal tissues, and possibly pain during sex. Testing will show no fungal elements present, which rules out a yeast infection. Bacterial and yeast infections can have similar symptoms, and it may be difficult to differentiate between them without a test. A disruption of balance in the vaginal flora leads to normally present bacteria either growing or decreasing in numbers, upsetting the pH and flora. In my clinical practice, I have seen a direct correlation between food issues and BV, particularly a high sugar intake. Clean up your diet by reducing sugars, simple carbohydrates, and alcohol. Be sure to stay hydrated.

SITZ BATH

This treatment will support your body against BV. See page 243 for more on sitz baths.

2 ounces (56 g) dried calendula flowers

2 ounces (56 g) dried echinacea root

1 ounce (28 g) dried yarrow flowers

YIELD: 4 ounces (112 g or about 6 baths)
Combine all ingredients in a bowl; store the mixture in a glass jar until needed. Infuse 6 tablespoons (27 g) in 1 quart (946 ml) of water overnight. Strain in the morning; save the herbs for another round of infusion. Gently warm the infusion and pour the liquid into your sitz bath basin. Sit down in the warm infusion for 15 minutes. Do 1 to 2 times daily for 3 to 5 days.

BACK OFF BV WASH

Bacterial vaginosis or yeast infections occur when the positive flora of the vagina decreases and overgrowth of negative bacteria or yeast rises. Release the stigma that you have done something wrong or bad, as either can arise spontaneously. There is no need for shame or self-sabotage. It is an opportunity to learn more about your body and how to care for it. I've had countless frustrated friends go to doctor after doctor, only to get another infection because the treatment they tried didn't work or only worked temporarily. You know your body better than anyone, and that includes your vagina. Get to know one another on a personal level. In many cultures, she is the center of your soul as a woman. I prefer washes to douches for the vagina. But you do you. If douches work better, go for it. Taking echinacea and yarrow tincture, in equal parts, internally at the same time is encouraged.

1 ounce (28 g) dried echinacea root

½ ounce (14 g) dried chickweed leaf

½ ounce (14 g) dried yarrow flower

10 drops tea tree essential oil

YIELD: 1 vaginal wash
Soak herbs in 1 pint (473 ml) of hot water overnight. Strain. Add essential oil and mix well.

Fill a basin with the brew and sit down in it. Use a washcloth to apply directly to the vagina, on the inside of the labia and introitus (opening of the vagina). Use gentle strokes. The mixture can be applied warm by gently heating it on the stove or applied cool. Apply twice daily for 5 days.

YEAST INFECTIONS

Not a bacterial infection, a yeast infection occurs when the flora of the vaginal canal is off, allowing the *Candida albicans* fungus to thrive. *Candida albicans* occurs normally within the body; it only becomes a problem when the balance is upset. Symptoms include burning, intense itching, swelling, discharge, and irritation of the vaginal tissue. Bringing about balance in the flora is the key to treatment. Simply killing off the fungus and not reestablishing the balance will only result in continued reoccurrence. Using probiotics internally and as suppositories is one way to help swing the pendulum back in favor of positive bacteria balance, which is necessary to keep yeast away. If you are experiencing chronic yeast infections, please seek guidance from a naturopathic physician who specializes in women's health.

YEAST AWAY WASH

Like to the BV Wash, this wash is formulated for yeast and overgrowth of fungal elements.

1 ounce (28 g) dried usnea lichen

1 ounce (28 g) dried goldenseal root

1 ounce (28 g) dried black walnut hull

10 drops tea tree essential oil

YIELD: 1 pint (473 ml)

Soak herbs in 1 pint (473 ml) of hot water overnight. Strain. Add 10 drops essential oil and mix well. Fill a basin with the brew and sit down in it. Use a washcloth to apply directly to the vagina, on the inside of the labia and introitus (opening of the vagina). Use gentle strokes. The mixture can be applied warm by gently heating it on the stove or applied cool. Apply twice daily for 5 days.

VARIATION: TREAT YOUR PARTNER TOO

If you are experiencing repeated infection, it is most likely your partner needs to be treated as well. Male or female, sometimes infection shows no signs. The treatment above and the BV Wash on page 113 can be applied to either sex. For men, simply soak a cotton cloth into the infusion and wrap the penis and testicles for a direct application. Leave on for 15 minutes.

ANTI-ITCH PACK

There is just no delicate way to speak of vaginal itching, is there? If you've experienced it, you know it's brutal and you'll do just about anything to find relief. This is a poultice mixed with yogurt for a cooling application when heat and itchiness are troubling you.

Pinch of dried lavender **Pinch of dried chickweed** **Pinch of dried elderflower** **1 teaspoon (5 g) cold yogurt**	**YIELD:** 1 pack Grind the herbs in your herb grinder. I use a cheap coffee grinder designated only for herbs. Add just enough hot water to turn the mixture into a paste. Add yogurt and mix. Apply inside the labia and leave on for 15 minutes or overnight. If wearing overnight, be sure to wear a pad. Whenever you are finished, wash clean with a cool, damp cloth.

VAGINAL WASH TO SOOTHE IRRITATION

Yogurt, tea tree oil, and garlic applications are well known to help with yeast infections. I also like a gentle wash using the following infusion to soothe inflamed tissues and provide healing relief.

½ ounce (14 g) dried calendula flowers **1 ounce (28 g) dried chickweed** **½ ounce (14 g) dried plantain leaf** **½ ounce (14 g) dried comfrey leaf** **½ ounce (14 g) dried roses**	**YIELD:** 3 ounces (84 g) Stir all herbs together; store in a glass jar. To make a wash, steep 4 tablespoons (18 g) herb mixture in 1 pint (475 ml) hot water for 2 to 3 hours or overnight; strain in the morning. Use a cotton cloth to drench the labia and external vaginal tissue.

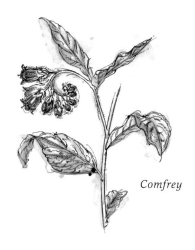

Comfrey

VAGINAL CAPSULES

To be inserted vaginally, these capsules help to decrease yeast overload and the symptoms associated with yeast infections.

¼ ounce (7 g) goldenseal powder	YIELD: 200 capsules
¼ ounce (7 g) myrrh powder	Mix all ingredients in a bowl; fill empty vegetable
1 ounce (28 g) boric acid powder	capsules with the mixture. Insert 2 capsules
½ ounce (14 g) slippery elm powder	vaginally each night for 7 days. Be sure to wear
	a pad while sleeping.

YEAST FREE TEA

Drink this tea for 2 to 4 weeks to work from the inside out. If yeast is pervading the digestive track, it can throw off the vaginal flora.

½ ounce (14 g) dried usnea lichen	YIELD: 2.5 ounces (70 g)
½ ounce (14 g) dried pau d'arco	Combine all ingredients; store in a glass jar.
¼ ounce (7 g) dried yarrow leaf and flower	Make medicinal strength (see page 245) and
¼ ounce (7 g) dried lavender flower	drink 3 cups daily.
1½ ounces (42 g) dried peppermint leaf	

BIRTH CONTROL

Let's chat a little about birth control. As easy as it is to gain access to birth control, I still find many young women confused about their options. The chart at right lists the different types of birth control currently available, according to Planned Parenthood. As we cling to the right to access birth control and our right to make choices for bodies, we need to exercise tolerance. As our world becomes more and more susceptible to whole groups of people being outcast due to their practices and beliefs, please attempt to practice compassion and peace for others who may believe differently than you do.

The recipes that follow the table are to help reestablish healthy reproductive function and hormonal balance after birth control is discontinued.

BIRTH CONTROL TYPE	FUNCTION
Breastfeeding as birth control	When you are breastfeeding exclusively, you are typically not ovulating, decreasing your chance of conception. But it is always best to use secondary protection.
Cervical cap	The cervical cap covers your cervix, preventing sperm from joining an egg entering the uterus. It is best used with spermicide.
Condom	Condoms are small, thin pouches made of latex, plastic, or lambskin that cover the penis during sex and collect semen. The condom's goal is to stop sperm from entering the vagina.
Diaphragm	The diaphragm is a barrier that covers your cervix; you bend it in half and insert it inside your vagina. It is best used with spermicide.
Female condoms	These cover the inside of your vagina, creating a barrier that stops sperm from entering the uterus. The female condom also helps prevent sexually transmitted infections.
Implant	Inserted under the skin of your upper arm, it releases the hormone progestin to prevent pregnancy.
Injection/Shot	Contains the hormone progestin, which stops ovulation; also works by thickening the cervical mucus.
IUD	A tiny device that's inserted in your uterus to prevent pregnancy. In theory, it acts as something already implanted in the uterus, preventing anything else from implanting. There are five types of IUDs: The first, Paragard, is also known as the Copper-T. The others, Mirena, Kyleena, Liletta, and Skyla, all use the hormone progestin to prevent pregnancy. Mirena works for up to 6 years, Kyleena up to 5 years, Liletta up to 4 years, and Skyla up to 3 years.
Patch	You wear the patch on certain parts of your body, and the hormones are absorbed through your skin. The patch stops your ovaries from releasing eggs and thickens the cervical mucus, which makes it hard for sperm to swim.
Pill	Stops ovulation and thickens the cervical mucus. Can be estrogen or progesterone based.
Sponge	Placed deep inside your vagina before sex. the sponge covers your cervix and contains spermicide to help prevent pregnancy. Each sponge has a fabric loop attached for easy removal.
Vaginal ring	The ring contains estrogen and progestin. You wear the ring inside your vagina, where the lining absorbs the hormones. It stops ovulation and thickens the cervical mucus.

BIRTH CONTROL COMEDOWN TONIC TEA

Drink this tea daily for 6 to 8 weeks to support the new hormonal normal for your body.

1½ ounces (42 g) dried burdock root	YIELD: 8 ounces (224 g)
1 ounce (28 g) dried alfalfa leaf	Combine ingredients; store in a glass jar.
1 ounce (28 g) dried motherwort leaf	Make medicinal strength (see page 245)
1 ounce (28 g) dried vitex berry	and drink 2 or 3 cups daily.
1 ounce (28 g) dried passionflower leaf	
1 ounce (28 g) dried chamomile flowers	
1½ ounces (42 g) dried lemon balm	

LET'S REESTABLISH BALANCE TINCTURE

Utilizing the natural hormonal ebb and flow, take this tincture upon rising in the morning to match the natural rise in cortisol.

2 tablespoons (30 ml) vitex berry tincture	YIELD: 2 ounces (60 ml)
2 teaspoons (10 ml) rhodiola root bark tincture	Combine all ingredients in a 2-ounce (60 ml)
2 teaspoons (10 ml) lady's mantle tincture	amber dropper bottle. Take 2 dropperfuls
2 teaspoons (10 ml) ginger root tincture	upon rising.

ESSENTIAL OIL BATH BLEND

Add 20 to 40 drops to your bath, depending on your scent preference, for a relaxing and supportive therapeutic soak.

1¼ teaspoons (6 ml) clary sage oil	YIELD: 2 teaspoons (10 ml)
½ teaspoon (3 ml) ylang-ylang oil	Combine oils; store in a 10 ml essential oil
½ teaspoon (3 ml) lavender oil	bottle.

ESCHAROTIC TREATMENT

I was introduced to escharotic treatment while working at what is now National University of Natural Medicine. This treatment is for those with diagnosed cervical dysplasia, which occurs when healthy cells of the cervix undergo changes due to trauma, infection, or disease, most commonly the human papillomavirus (HPV), a sexually transmitted disease with hundreds of different strains. It's typically diagnosed during a Pap test, for which some cells are taken from the surface of the cervix and examined microscopically. Initial suspicion of cervical dysplasia can be based on a visual examination of the cervix and a colposcopy exam can confirm diagnosis. This condition is most often benign, but it can lead to cervical cancer, particularly when certain genetic markers are present.

The following description of escharotic treatment is for educational purposes only. It must be performed by a clinically trained professional as self-performing could damage cervical tissue. Patients are generally seen twice per week for five to six weeks. While the patient rests in the obstetrical position, a speculum is inserted into the vaginal canal. First, powdered bromelain is applied to the cervix and a warming light is shined upon the cervical area for fifteen minutes. The bromelain powder is then removed with cotton-tipped applicators that have been soaked in calendula succus, raw herb juice that is extremely beneficial for wound care.

Next, a mixture of zinc chloride and herbal tincture of bloodroot (*Sanguinaria canadensis*) is applied and left on for one minute. Then the cervix is wiped clean with cotton-tipped applicators soaked in calendula succus. Finally, two vegetable capsules filled with vaginal supportive herbs and homeopathics is inserted close to the cervix. Treatment continues at home with oral and vaginal suppositories of herbal/homeopathic supplements.

These are the treatment options available for cervical dysplasia and HPV. I have seen firsthand the healing effects of this treatment and find it to be much less invasive than the typical approach of cutting and incising the cervix. By supporting and targeting the area, there is hope for returning health and healing to these precious tissues.

Dawning can be an empowering time if you choose to honor and celebrate it. Moving through life understanding the changes your body is going through as well as how it works gives you power. Take time to think about all that is going on in your life during this time. Being a young woman only happens once, and it goes faster than you think. Harness the power you possess and ride the lightening you create.

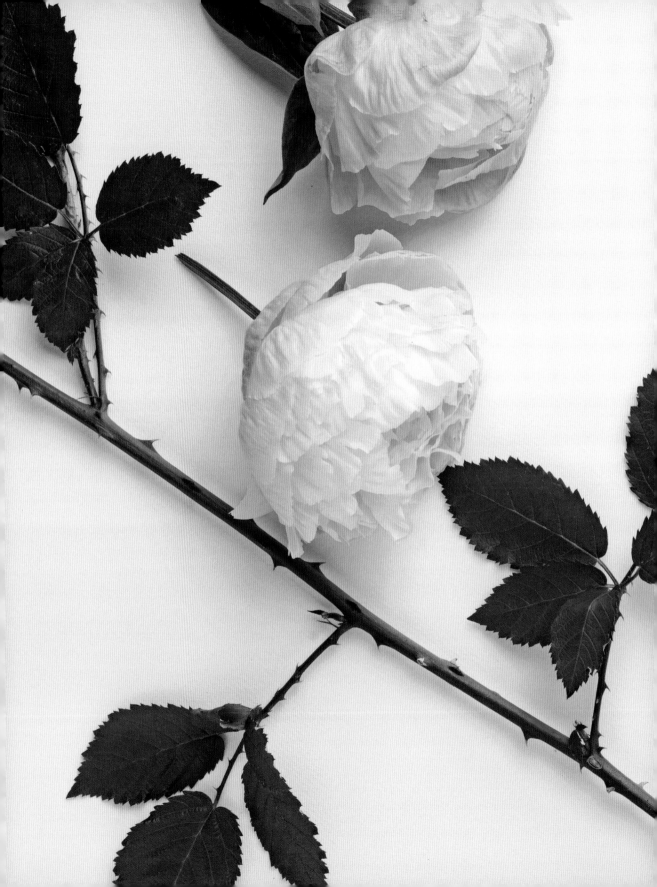

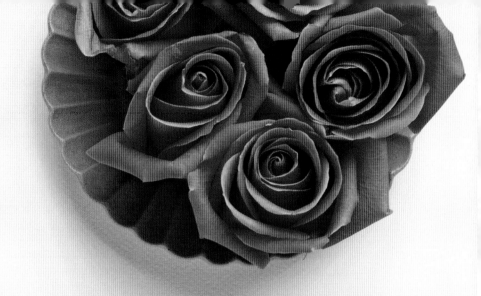

CHAPTER 4

Living
Twenties to Perimenopause

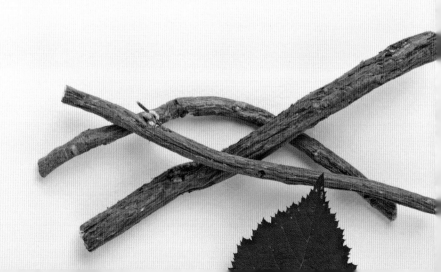

LIVING is the time frame from your twenties to the close of your reproductive years. You are moving through your days with intention, new directions, ideas, and creation. You are hopeful, and the dreams of your future are almost tangible. Your body is heightened in form and function, ready to adjust and compensate for everything you do. Your central nervous system, heart, digestion, and hormonal processes are at their height of function. Your liver is capable of handling almost anything that comes its way, making detoxification thorough and complete. Stress is still moderated by the adrenal glands, and optimal physical function is easier to achieve. Although youth has a way of making you feel invincible, know that how you take care of your body now will determine how well it functions in the years to come.

Living is the phase that most of my interns, staff, and new herbal students are in when I meet them. I refer to them as the herbal-enthusiastic youth who are reclaiming their bodies and the wisdom of herbal medicine. Perhaps you too are reading this and feeling the excitement of what herbs and herbal medicine have to offer. Maybe with each page you read, you are remembering the connection to plants you had as child—for instance, when you climbed a tree, picked a pretty flower, or joyfully played in the grass. You remember the sense of healing and connection to your body that nature offered. Remembering the feelings connected to plants and the healing they offer gives you hope and connection to yourself and your body. Time and time again, I hear the same story from new herb students. They say it's as though they already know the information when they learn about the herbs and their potential. For many, it's a natural transition into using herbs regularly.

As we reach our twenties, we have gained experience and knowledge about ourselves and our bodies. We typically know what works for our bodies and what doesn't, even if we haven't mastered how to consistently choose correctly. A helpful concept to consider for the Living phase is the theory of the seven-year health cycle for women. It has been studied by many healing philosophies, including Chinese medicine and biodynamic emotional healing practitioners. Using a framework of human development in seven-year increments can teach us what about our bodies is growing, being developed, or in decline depending on where we are in our life. Such insight gives us the opportunity to use herbal medicine to support wherever we are in our life cycle. By working with the body's natural cycles, we can feel and be our best any stage of life. The Living cycle flows through the reproductive years, when many women decide to conceive and have children. Knowing this cycle is helpful when considering conception and caring for children.

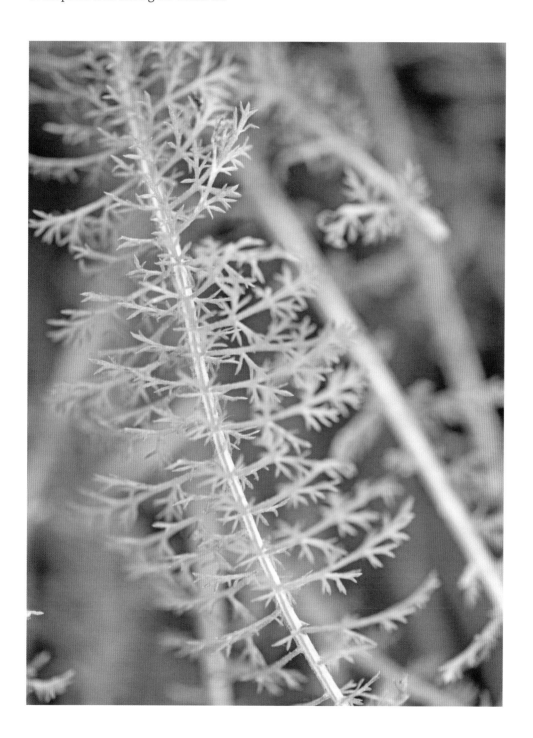

THE ENERGETIC THEORY OF THE CYCLES
OF THE FEMALE

Cycle One

The first cycle begins at birth and is complete at age seven. Our growth and sustainability are focused on basic needs of care, food, and love. These are the foundations of survival. The first organs to be completely developed in utero are the kidneys, because processing nutrients and eliminating waste are necessary for survival. According to Chinese medicine philosophy, at the time of conception some energy (known as *jing*) is taken from both the mother and the father to create the child. The health of this energy is dependent on how healthy the parents are. If both parents are relatively healthy, there is adequate energy to spare, and the child starts off balanced and in good health. If they are not, the child may start life deficient in energy, which can cause initial developmental struggles or weakened health at any time of life.

As we continue to make strides in the field of genetics, you can also think of the word *energy* as genetics. As we now know, genes and their expression can be turned on or off depending on the state of our health. Another way to conceptualize this is to think of this energy as a person's constitution. I'm sure you've heard the saying "She has a strong constitution." The prenatal energy is the constitution, the foundation. What happens to children after birth is the accumulation of postnatal energy. This is gained through what they eat, the love they receive, the conditions they live in, and their overall health. All this postnatal energy contributes to the health of the child and eventually the adult. As I mentioned above, the kidneys filter out waste and retain nutrients. In essence, the kidneys train us to hold onto what is vital and release what is not. Being able to do this is important throughout life.

Using herbs throughout the first seven years not only supports the developing systems of the body but also creates nourishment in a unique way. Children use an exorbitant amount of energy on a daily basis. Ensuring they have all the nutrients they need to reach their fullest potential can be challenging. Herbal syrups, teas, and glycerin drops offer additional options when eating regularly becomes a struggle. With my daughter, tea parties became a regular occurrence beginning at age two. Having tea as a normal part of her routine made it easy to incorporate it into her diet when needed. For example, when she was "too busy" to eat and I didn't feel like battling to get her to, we'd compromise on tea. I would make her a cup of mineral tea: alfalfa, nettle leaf, dandelion leaf, barley, and a bit of honey. Not ideal, but as any parent can attest, it's better than nothing when your kid just won't eat. Each spring I'd make a nettle leaf, dandelion root, and catnip syrup to support her liver and digestive system. It's not that anything was wrong, but the energy of spring is a great time to support the liver, and supporting the liver and digestive system is doing what I do best—preventive medicine. Another great way to use herbs with kids is herbal candy. You can mix different combinations of powdered herbs with honey and nut butter. Simply roll this mixture into little balls and store them in the refrigerator.

From ages seven to fourteen, a whole new world begins to form around children. They will often start to explore outside their normal comfort zone and be able to do things physically that they weren't able to do before. On the inside, their kidneys are now vital and strong. New systems are getting more development attention. As the body grows, the sense of self, what a child likes and doesn't, also grows. The opportunity for independent thinking increases, and the reproductive system is slowly coming into maturation. Hair, teeth, and bones are also growing stronger. Baby teeth are often lost around ages six and seven, a sign that a child is vital and healthy. According to educational theorist, social reformer, and philosopher Rudolph Steiner, the loss of teeth indicates a shift in focus away from body awareness to the beginning of mental capacity. One example of this is the shift from kindergarten, which is often focused on play, to first-grade brain learning, such as reading and math.

This is a wonderful time to introduce children to herbs and making herbal medicine. I often start with teaching them how to make a lip balm or a salve. Most children enjoy hands-on activities that result in an end product they can use. Having the lip balm after making it themselves can inspire them. Teaching them how to make tea and encouraging them to blend different herbs together makes for a fun afternoon as you try out different mixtures. As with anything you do with kids, give them the keys for success. Use herbs such as mint, chamomile, catnip, lemon balm, rose petals, and lavender, which all have a relatively pleasant flavor. Growing up with herbs as a part of their home medicine gives children an advantage as they age. They are often more knowledgeable and confident in caring for themselves as adults.

Cycle Two

The next cycle begins at age fourteen, and the most apparent development is in the reproductive organs. If they haven't already, girls often are experiencing menarche, hormone regulation, and breast development. Again referring to Chinese medicine philosophy, a girl's energy and blood are strong at this age, and her capabilities are limitless if given the opportunity. From the ages of fourteen to twenty-one, girls are experiencing an extremely important time of physical, emotional, and mental development. Because she is young, her physical health is often vital even if her resources are less than ideal. The impact of what her surroundings offer will be profound at this time and have the potential to shape who she will become. If she is given a positive opportunity, a positive environment, and/or the knowledge of how to communicate and express herself, she will have an incredible foundation for her future. Young women at this stage have a growing need to create personal and private space. Seeking self-identity within the world they've known their whole life—primarily the family unit—balanced with developing their identity in the outside world via dating, expanded social activities, and school can make this stage overwhelming and confusing to a young woman. Using herbs to support her menstrual cycle and emotional well-being will not only ease this cycle but also help encourage healthy cycles for years to come.

Cycle Three

At the exciting age of twenty-one, young women are often living busy lives, and their fertility energy is considered fully developed. Ovulation and menstruation are typically well established. Cultures around the world picture *the maiden* as a young, round, soft woman aged twenty-one to twenty-eight. I like to use the word *full* because it encompasses what this time offers her. Fertility, or being fertile, gives us the perception of being full. But it's not just a physical fullness; she is also full of dreams, creations, and hopes for the future. I often hear of young women who don't wish to get pregnant having birthing dreams at this age. A pregnancy or baby dream often indicates the creation of something new in one's life. Philosopher Tony Crisp says it so well: We start to build the foundations of our careers and intimate relationships with a driving energy that we hope will gain us entry and respect in the larger world. Perhaps a young woman has just started working full-time, has taken on the responsibility of a new project, or has made a relationship commitment to another person. These are all new steps into adulthood and are the defining nonphysical aspects for this time.

Drink herbal teas daily to support your life during this phase. If you notice something out of rhythm, try to identify it. Ask yourself questions and do your best to determine what might be causing the change you feel. Try using herbs in new ways, perhaps as tinctures or syrups. Ensuring your reproductive and digestive systems are balanced and functioning well throughout this time will promote health down the road.

Whatever routines you establish from ages twenty-one to twenty-seven will create who you are at twenty-eight. Try your best to have regular exercise, positive outlets for fun, and balanced eating habits. At twenty-one years old, I ate a lot of ramen noodles and McDonalds. I was poor, and these foods were easy and cheap. No one really taught me how to cook as a child, but when I moved to Seattle at age twenty-five, I was determined to try. I remember walking around the produce section in awe of the number of vegetables I had never seen before. I chose kale and beets to take home with me. Although the first several attempts at cooking them weren't very tasty, I definitely felt better after eating them than I did after eating a meal from McDonalds. By age twenty-eight, I had two years of cooking disasters and successes under my belt. (One downside to being poor is that even if what you cook tastes awful, you have to eat it!)

Cycle Four

Age twenty-eight is a good time to take a moment and reflect on your physical health. If you are experiencing a physical symptom regularly, it's time to explore practitioner-guided care. This could mean headaches, digestive upset, insomnia, menstrual irregularities—basically anything that is a deviation of normal function. I'm continually surprised at what woman consider normal these days. Having a headache twice a week isn't normal, folks. Seek health care and get some relief. Many of us learn to live with daily health inconveniences without realizing they can change. The first step is to achieve body awareness and become the expert in how and what affects your body. When does the symptom occur? What makes it worse? Better? Pay attention and be your own health detective.

Cycle Five

At ages twenty-eight to thirty-six, we're often faced with a persistent desire to create change if change is needed. This could be a small change in your routine or diet or a big change in your relationship or job. If the winds of change are calling, I urge you to follow your heart. Remember, you can always come back. The cost of not listening to what needs to be changed in your life will take its toll over time.

Use herbs to help you feel your best and to help you see clearly what you want for yourself. When your body is free of toxins, your brain thinks without resistance and your heart can guide you to your truth. Establish supportive herbal routines. Perhaps each month you might focus on one area of your body, such as the heart, hormones, or respiratory system. Have a daily tea or tincture to support whichever system you are working with. Use herbs in ceremony as you work through what is and what isn't working in your life. Reflect upon the moon and sip on rosemary and damiana to entice your dreams to share the secrets of your subconscious.

I remember being a young child and thinking that thirty-five was so old! But as a woman of thirty-five, you have often reached a whole new level of self-empowerment and physical strength. This is the age at which it is important to begin regular self-care of the physical body. Self-care is also considered preventive care. Care for your skin by washing and moisturizing regularly. Care for your heart and circulatory system with regular cardiovascular exercise and dry skin brushing. Care for your soul with scheduled massages, facials, or a walk in your favorite woods. This is an interesting age, and it is the time I often see new patients in my office. I call it the "all of a sudden" phase, because symptoms see to arise out of nowhere. This is when I educate the patient on how the body works. It isn't that all things suddenly quit working; it's more that you've reached a tipping point and the body now must pick and choose which areas to focus on. Symptoms tend to arise in the areas that are now getting less attention.

A common example is a new food allergy. A patient may come in complaining that suddenly she can no longer eat cheese without gas and bloating. Nine times out of ten, the patient's body has always struggled to digest cheese but was able to compensate for years. As the body ages, it can no longer make such compensations. As inflammation increases, the digestive system loses its ability to digest properly. As a result, new symptoms arise.

Another example is the rise in insomnia as we age. In Chinese medicine philosophy, sometime between the ages of thirty-five and forty-two is when your energy resources begin to dissipate. This means that unless you do healthy things to fill up the reserves, aging has the potential to accelerate. If you've had stress in your life for a while and haven't done anything to replenish yourself, your adrenal glands have most likely been overexerted. Over time, one of the side effects of the adrenals losing their reserves is ineffective cortisol release. This can affect sleep patterns. If you make healthy living a priority, you can perpetually fill up your vital energy and decrease the aging process.

My top tips to accomplish this?

1. Hydrate.

2. Eat loads of vegetables daily.

3. Drink teas made with nourishing tonic herbs.

4. Exercise.

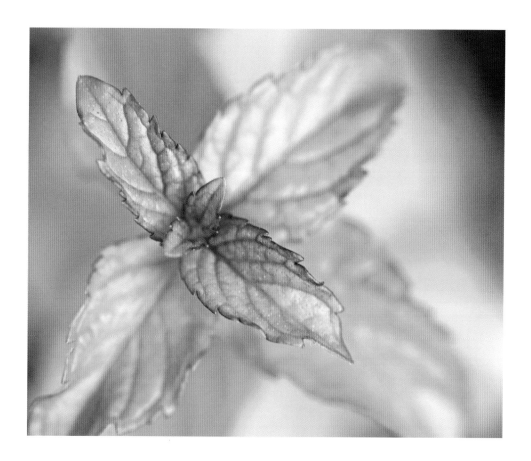

THE LIVING PHASE

The entire Living phase is a prime opportunity to use herbs to promote health and healing. I've also found that learning and using herbs at this time of your life creates a deeper connection to your body. Those who begin their herbal journey during the Living phase will, more often than not, use herbs again and again throughout their lives.

It's important to create balance during the Living phase. If you are experiencing obvious hormonal imbalance, now is the time to address it. The earlier we course correct hormones, the easier it is. The longer you wait, the longer it takes to shift the body back into balance. Looking into your future, think about caring for your body like a temple. Honor it and care for it, and it will provide for you.

From the ages of twenty-one to forty-two, one woman can be lucky and sail through on the winds of health while another will struggle with symptoms of imbalance. The conditions I see most commonly during the Living phase are fibroids, ovarian cysts, PCOS, endometriosis, heavy bleeding, fertility and conception concerns, pregnancy, and postpartum issues. Bladder complaints, stress, general fatigue, and other topics are included in the "Support" chapter of this book. Many women also experience menstrual irregularity, spotting, and PMS during this phase, so please see the "Dawning" chapter, as these are covered there.

As a doctor, woman, and friend, I've had many personal conversations about pregnancy. I feel strongly that it is every woman's choice to have children or not. The decision to have children, no matter how many, is a personal choice, just as is the decision to not have children. Woman live powerfully fulfilled lives in either case and should not be judged for the choices that best reflect who they are and what they want in life. To lift up our womankind, be kind and not judgmental regarding the choices others make.

With each of the following conditions, I will provide easy recipes for making your own herbal medicine at home. As a reminder, herbs are powerful medicine and always need to be used with knowledge and wisdom.

Common Physical Complaints of the Living Phase

Fibroids	Heavy bleeding	Labor support
Ovarian issues	Fertility	Postpartum
Endometriosis	Pregnancy	

FIBROIDS

Let's just say it: Fibroids are annoying. They are one of the first "diagnoses" that may women encounter, often identified during an annual physical exam when they are not even aware of them. If untreated, fibroids can grow and eventually lead to increased menstrual bleeding, pregnancy implantation issues, pain during sex, backache, and digestive issues. Although benign, meaning they aren't cancerous and rarely become cancerous, they are frustrating. No one should have to suffer through any of their symptoms, and sex should be pleasurable, not painful. The one consideration with herbal treatment of fibroids is that there is minimal success in completely shrinking those of significant size. There is noted success with inhibiting growth and greatly reducing smaller fibroids, but both require diligence and consistent treatment as part of daily life.

There are three types of fibroids: submucosal, intramural, and subserosal. Submucosal fibroids grow into the uterus. They can take up space in the uterine cavity, cause heavy bleeding, and interfere with conception. Intramural fibroids grow between the inside and outside of the uterus, actually in the uterine muscle. Subserosal fibroids grow on the outside of the uterus, where they can often be felt during an abdominal/uterine exam.

Determining the cause of fibroids can be complicated because it is most likely more than one element. In today's world, women are subjected to much more that affects our bodies and hormones than in previous decades. Phthalates, xenoestrogens, food preservatives, higher stress loads, poorer water quality, some types of birth control, lack of estrogen, African-American decent, and prolonged sitting have all been linked to fibroids.

In addition to the recipes that follow, you might consider some other natural treatments as well. Refer to chapter 1 for details on each.

- Digestive enzymes between meals; the idea is that the enzymes will target the fibroid and aid in breakdown.
- Mayan abdominal massage to reduce pelvic stagnation.
- Acupuncture and moxa to reduce pelvic stagnation.

Stock your herbal pantry with the following for fibroids:

Black Cohosh root	Ginger root	Shepherd's Purse
Burdock root	Licorice root	Turmeric root
Cinnamon bark	Nettle leaf	Vitex berry
Dandelion root	Orange peel	Wild Yam root
Fennel seed	Oregon Grape root	Yellow Dock root

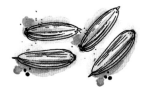

Fennel

TEA TO HALT FIBROID GROWTH

I've yet to see herbal medicine alone completely dissolve uterine fibroids, but I have had some success with inhibiting growth.

2 ounces (56 g) dried burdock root	YIELD: 8 ounces (224 g)
1 ounce (28 g) dried dandelion root	Combine all ingredients; store in a glass
¾ ounce (21 g) dried yellow dock root	jar. Make medicinal strength (see page
1 ounce (28 g) dried Oregon grape root	245) and drink 3 cups daily for 12 weeks.
1 ounce (28 g) dried wild yam root	
¼ ounce (7 g) dried ginger root	
1½ ounces (42 g) dried orange peel	
¾ ounce (21 g) dried fennel seed	

FIBROID GROWTH HALTER TINCTURE

Here's another optional treatment to consolidate efforts to stop fibroid growth.

Note: Replace licorice root with 1 tablespoon (15 ml) rhodiola and 1 tablespoon (15 ml) of slippery elm bark if you have hypertension.

2 tablespoons (30 ml) black cohosh root tincture	YIELD: 4 ounces (120 ml)
1½ tablespoon (25 ml) licorice root tincture	Combine all ingredients in a 4-ounce
1½ tablespoon (25 ml) vitex berry tincture	(120 ml) amber dropper bottle. Take 2
1½ tablespoon (25 ml) turmeric root tincture	dropperfuls 3 times per day between meals
1 tablespoon (15 ml) nettle leaf tincture	for 8 to 12 weeks. Do not take with food.

EXCESSIVE BLEEDING TINCTURE

Sometimes fibroids can cause excessive menstrual bleeding. If you are noticing flooding, or prolonged bleeding, give this tincture a try.

4 teaspoons (20 ml) shepherd's purse tincture	YIELD: 1 ounce (28 ml)
2 teaspoons (10 ml) cinnamon bark tincture	Combine all ingredients in a 1-ounce (28 ml) amber dropper bottle.
	DOSAGE: 1 to 2 dropperfuls every 20 minutes until bleeding greatly reduces; not to exceed 6 to 8 doses per 24 hours.

FIBROID HORMONE BALANCE TINCTURE

This hormonal tonic targets fibroids and the excess hormones that often create them.

2 tablespoons (30 ml) burdock root tincture	YIELD: 4 ounces (120 ml)
2 tablespoons (30 ml) vitex berry tincture	Combine all ingredients in a 4-ounce (120 ml) amber dropper bottle.
1 tablespoon (15 ml) black cohosh root tincture	Take 1 dropperful 3 times per day for 8 to 12 weeks.
1 tablespoon (15 ml) wild yam root tincture	
1½ teaspoons (7.5 ml) dandelion root tincture	
1½ teaspoons (7.5 ml) yellow dock root tincture	
1½ teaspoons (7.5 ml) Oregon grape root tincture	
1½ teaspoons (7.5 ml) ginger root tincture	

ESSENTIAL OIL BLEND

This blend is to be used topically on the abdomen over the uterus in an effort to reduce fibroid growth.

50 drops cypress essential oil	YIELD: 2 teaspoons (10 ml)
50 drops frankincense essential oil	Combine all oils in a 5 ml glass European essential oil dropper bottle. Rub a small amount on the abdomen over the uterus each night for 4 to 6 weeks.
25 drops basil essential oil	
15 drops thyme essential oil	
½ teaspoon (3 ml) apricot essential oil	

OVARY ISSUES

Our ovaries direct our reproductive hormones and process in a delicate dance every month. Supporting their function and the hormones that influence them is one way to improve reproductive health.

Stock your home herbal pantry with the following for ovarian health:

Alfalfa leaf	Corn Silk	Poke root
Blue Cohosh	Crampbark	Slippery Elm bark
Burdock root	Gravel root	Vitex berry
Chamomile flowers	Nettle leaf	White Peony
Chickweed	Peppermint leaf	Wormwood

Ovarian Cysts

These painful fluid-filled sacks arise on the ovaries and can grow to impressive size. Some grow and shrink each month with the hormone fluctuations; others grow and grow until bursting. I've had many patients end up in the Emergency Room with intense pain from ovarian cyst rupture. This pain is severe, and I would never question a woman's discomfort in such a situation.

HERBAL INFUSED CASTOR OIL

Topical application is one way to treat any condition. Castor oil's anti-inflammatory actions pair well with the following herbs to reduce pain and occurrence of ovarian cysts.

1 ounce (28 g) dried chickweed

1 ounce (28 g) dried crampbark

½ ounce (14 g) dried poke root

16 ounces (475 ml) castor oil

8 ounces (235 ml) olive oil

YIELD: 1 to 2 cups (235 to 475 ml)

Preheat oven to 170°F (77°C). In a glass baking dish, cover herbs with castor and olive oils. Bake for 4 hours. Strain and store in a container of your choice. Apply 1 to 3 teaspoons (5 to 15 ml) twice daily to the abdomen above the ovaries.

HORMONES TARGETED: OVARIAN CYSTS

Reducing estrogen levels and pain, as well as supporting optimal ovarian function, is the focus of this blend.

3 tablespoons (45 ml) vitex berry tincture	YIELD: 4 ounces (120 ml)
3 tablespoons (45 ml) blue cohosh root tincture	Combine all ingredients in a 4-ounce (120 ml) amber dropper bottle. Take 1 dropperful 3 times per day.
3 tablespoons (45 ml) white peony root tincture	

POTASSIUM BLAST TEA

Theories abound that cysts are easily created when potassium is deficient. This tea will provide some needed potassium to make it more difficult for them to form.

1 ounce (28 g) dried corn silk	YIELD: 8 ounces (224 g)
1 ounce (28 g) dried nettle	Combine all ingredients; store in a glass jar. Make medicinal strength (see page 245) and drink 2 cups daily for 4 to 8 weeks.
1 ounce (28 g) dried alfalfa	
2 ounces (56 g) dried burdock	
3 ounces (84 g) dried peppermint	

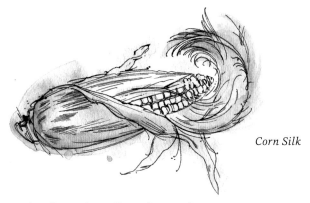

Corn Silk

PCOS (Polycystic Ovarian Syndrome)

PCOS is diagnosed when a woman shows multiple cysts on an ovary or ovaries. This can happen due to hormone imbalance, ovary dysfunction, or the use of birth control. The symptoms can vary, but the most common are menstrual irregularities, absence of menstrual cycle, acne, weight gain around the middle, excessive hair loss or growth, fertility issues, mood disorders, and/or blood sugar/insulin disorder. Treatments that get the ovary back to regular function are best.

PCOS TINCTURE

This was the formula I was prescribed when I was diagnosed with PCOS. It was my first experience with herbal tinctures, and I'll never forget it. The taste was intense, but my body began to crave it. Although I also utilized acupuncture, made dietary changes, and stopped smoking, I know this tincture did its part in reestablishing my ovulation function.

⅓ cup (80 ml) vitex berry tincture

3 tablespoons (45 ml) false unicorn root (*Chamaelirium luteum*) tincture

YIELD: 4 ounces (120 ml)

Pour both herbal tinctures into a 4-ounce (120 ml) amber bottle; shake gently to mix. Take 1 teaspoon (5 ml) twice daily for 8 to 12 weeks.

TOPICAL OIL FOR PCOS

Combine the following oils for topical application. Utilizing both essential oils and herbal oils, this blend strives to regulate hormones that support natural ovulatory function.

½ ounce (14 g) dried motherwort leaf

½ ounce (14 g) dried cleavers leaf

1 cup (235 ml) olive oil

4 ounces (120 ml) castor oil

20 drops clary sage essential oil

10 drops geranium essential oil

10 drops ylang-ylang essential oil

10 drops lavender essential oil

YIELD: 1 cup (235 ml)

Preheat oven to 170°F (77°C). Place herbs in a glass baking dish and pour enough olive and castor oils over them to cover by 1 to 2 inches (3 to 5 cm). Bake for 4 hours. Allow to cool, and then strain into a storage container. Add essential oils and shake gently. Apply daily to the abdomen over the ovaries.

PCOS CAPSULE SUPPORT

If capsules are your preference, these are for you. They support ovarian function, with the added benefit of working through the digestive track, which is often compromised in PCOS patients.

1 ounce (28 g) vitex berry powder

¼ ounce (7 g) wild yam root powder

¼ ounce (7 g) yellow dock root powder

¼ ounce (7 g) Oregon grape root powder

¼ ounce (7 g) blue vervain leaf powder

YIELD: 200 capsules

Mix all ingredients in a bowl. Use the mixture to fill empty vegetable capsules. Take 2 capsules twice daily for 6 to 12 weeks.

ENDOMETRIOSIS

Endometriosis is a complicated disease that can have devastating effects on a woman. This condition can be limited to the reproductive organs, or it can make its way to almost any organ it chooses when left to its own devices. Pain is the key symptom here: worsening pain with menstruation, bowel pain, or pain with sex. Because many other conditions present similarly, prompt diagnosis is important and is often accomplished by pelvic examination and or ultrasound/scanning.

Stock your home herbal pantry with the following for endometriosis:

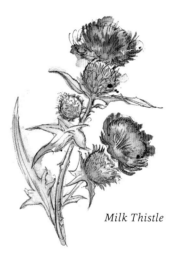

Burdock root	Plantain
Dandelion root	Poplar buds (fresh)
Dong Quai	Prickly Ash
Elderberry	Red Raspberry
Hawthorn berry	Saw Palmetto berry
Horsetail	St. John's Wort
Milk Thistle	Turmeric
Motherwort	Vitex berry

Milk Thistle

GENTLE MOVER TINCTURE

When we think of endometriosis, we often think of stagnation. This blend works to gently move the blood to reduce adhesions and pain. If you are experiencing excessive bleeding, try this formula in small doses initially. You may need to leave out the dong quai and motherwort because they move blood so well, but in the small amounts here, I find them more helpful to leave in. If you notice an increase in menstrual bleeding, replace them with 4 teaspoons (20 ml) of red clover.

2 tablespoons (30 ml) prickly ash bark tincture

4 teaspoons (20 ml) elderberry tincture

4 teaspoons (20 ml) blueberry tincture

4 teaspoons (20 ml) milk thistle tincture

2 teaspoons (10 ml) dong quai root tincture

2 teaspoons (10 ml) motherwort tincture

2 teaspoons (10 ml) dandelion root tincture

YIELD: 4 ounces (120 ml)

Combine all ingredients in a 4-ounce (120 ml) amber dropper bottle.

Take 1 dropperful 3 times per day.

TOPICAL ABDOMINAL CARE FOR ENDOMETRIOSIS

Using castor oil to reduce inflammation can significantly alleviate the discomforts of endometriosis. As previously discussed, the castor oil is absorbed through the skin; when herbally infused, it can possibly provide potent healing.

16 ounces (475 ml) castor oil

8 ounces (235 ml) olive oil

1 ounce (28 g) fresh horsetail leaf

½ ounce (14 g) fresh plantain leaf

1 ounce (28 g) St. John's wort flowers (fresh)

1 ounce (28 g) poplar buds (fresh)

YIELD: 3 cups (705 ml)

Place all ingredients in a slow cooker and set on low for 1 week. Strain mixture and store in an amber glass bottle. Apply twice daily to the abdomen.

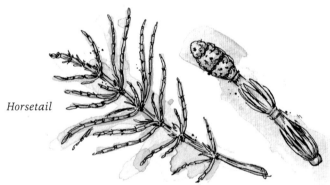

Horsetail

THE WOMAN'S HERBAL APOTHECARY

ENDOMETRIAL ANTI-INFLAMMATORY SUPPORT CAPSULES

These capsules are another herbal approach to reducing inflammation and endometrial clot formations that can lead to the adhesions of endometriosis.

½ ounce (14 g) saw palmetto berry powder

½ ounce (14 g) turmeric root powder

¼ ounce (7 g) prickly ash bark powder

¼ ounce (7 g) burdock root powder

YIELD: 100 capsules

Mix all ingredients in a bowl. Fill empty vegetable capsules with the mixture. Take 4 capsules twice daily.

MENORRHAGIA (HEAVY BLEEDING)

Whether you are experiencing a prolonged menstruation cycle or an excessive menstrual cycle, you need to reduce flow. Excessive bleeding can result in vitamin and mineral deficiencies, anemia, shortness of breath, and fatigue.

Stock your home herbal pantry with the following for heavy bleeding:

Blue Cohosh root	Crampbark	Motherwort
Cayenne	Ginger	Shepherd's Purse
Cinnamon	Mistletoe leaf	

MENORRHAGIA INHIBITOR TINCTURE

Heavy menstrual bleeding can leave you exhausted and weak. When enough is enough, reach for this herbal hemostatic.

⅓ cup (80 ml) shepherd's purse leaf tincture	**YIELD:** 4 ounces (120 ml)
2 tablespoons (30 ml) blue cohost root tincture	Combine all ingredients in a 4-ounce (120 m) amber dropper bottle.
2 teaspoons (10 ml) cinnamon bark tincture	Take 1 to 2 dropperfuls every 20 minutes for up to 4 hours to decrease or stop menstrual bleeding.
10 drops cayenne tincture	

SHOCK TEA (Courtesy: Dr. John Christopher)

Dr. John Christopher, an herbalist and naturopathic physician, made herbal medicine his lifelong study. His accounts of treating various people and conditions are amazing, and I've used this formula often to nip excessive menstrual bleeding in the bud.

1 cup (235 ml) warm water	**YIELD:** 1 serving
2 tablespoons (40 g) honey	Stir all ingredients together; drink.
1 tablespoon (15 ml) apple cider vinegar	
1 teaspoon (5 ml) cayenne powder	

139

HEADY DAYS TEA

Usually at some point in your menstrual bleeding, there are 1 to 2 heavier days. Drink this tea the day before and throughout those days to decrease excessive blood loss.

1 ounce (28 g) dried mistletoe leaf

1 ounce (28 g) dried blue cohosh root

1 ounce (28 g) dried crampbark

1 ounce (28 g) dried ginger root

YIELD: 4 ounces (112 g)

Combine all ingredients in a glass jar. Use to make tea as needed.

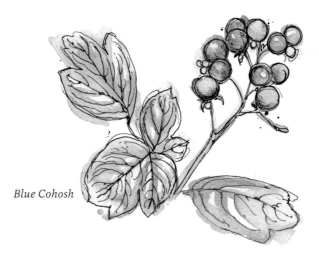

Blue Cohosh

CALM BLEEDING FOMENTATION

Sometimes a little self-care can go a long way. Use this poultice on heavy cramping/bleeding days to provide relief and reduction for both.

1 ounce (28 g) dried shepherd's purse leaf

1 ounce (28 g) dried saw palmetto berry

1 ounce (28 g) dried crampbark

1 ounce (28 g) dried mistletoe leaf

¼ ounce (7 g) dried cinnamon chips

YIELD: 1 treatment

Mix all ingredients. Place 8 tablespoons (36 g) in a muslin bag. Submerge in 4 cups (950 ml) of water and simmer on low, covered, for 30 minutes. Turn off the heat and let sit, covered, for another 30 minutes. Saturate a cotton cloth and place on your abdomen for 15 to 30 minutes covered with a warm towel.

FERTILITY

Truth be told, this section could be a whole book unto itself. There are so many helpful ways in which herbs can support the woman from conception to postpartum. The history of herbs in pregnancy is profound, and the gentle ways in which herbs can work truly support every woman through this rite of passage.

Stock your home herbal pantry with the following for fertility:

Alfalfa leaf

Angelica root

Black Cohosh

Burdock root

Chamomile

Dong Quai root

Ginger root

Kelp powder

Licorice root

Maca root

Oat Straw

Partridgeberry

Passionflower

Peppermint

Rose petals

Sassafras bark

Schizandra berry

Skullcap

Spirulina powder

Vitex berry

Wild Yam root

See the Dawning chapter for hormone regulation support to normalize menstrual cycles. If it doesn't happen quickly or easily, trying to conceive can switch from an exciting time to one filled with stress. Unfortunately, this raises hormones that inhibit conception. Supporting the reproductive system with hormone-balancing herbs and ensuring stress levels remain low are important. This is easier said than done; I myself experienced challenges when trying to conceive my second child. If your mind begins to take over, drink the Calm Vessel Tea (see next page) and do your best to stay positive.

FERTILITY TEA

This blend is packed with fertility-loving herbs.

2 ounces (56 g) dried vitex berry	YIELD: 10 ounces (280 g)
2 ounces (56 g) dried burdock root	Combine all ingredients; store in a
1 ounce (28 g) dried angelica root	glass jar. Make medicinal strength
1 ounce (28 g) dried dong quai root	overnight (see page 245) or simmer
1 ounce (28 g) dried sassafras bark	1 to 2 teaspoons (1.5 to 3 g) in 12 ounces
1 ounce (28 g) dried licorice root	(355 ml) of water, covered, on low for
1 ounce (28 g) dried orange peel	10 to 15 minutes. Strain and drink 3 cups
½ ounce (14 g) dried ginger root	per day for 6 to 12 weeks to prime your
½ ounce (14 g) dried black cohosh	body for conception.
½ ounce (14 g) dried wild yam root	

HAPPY OVARIES CAPSULES

Ensuring that our ovaries are getting the nutrients they need is just as important as having our hormones in check.

½ ounce (14 g) maca root powder

½ ounce (14 g) vitex berry powder

¼ ounce (7 g) spirulina powder

¼ ounce (7 g) kelp powder

¼ ounce (7 g) dong quai root powder

¼ ounce (7 g) schizandra berry powder

YIELD: 200 capsules

Combine all ingredients; use mixture to fill empty vegetable capsules. Take 2 capsules, 3 times per day.

THE DESTRESSED CONCEPTION TINCTURE

Trying to make a baby should be a fun and exciting time. Keep things in perspective and take this tincture daily to help support the emotional process.

2 tablespoons (30 ml) partridgeberry tincture

2 tablespoons (30 ml) skullcap tincture

4 teaspoons (20 ml) chamomile tincture

4 teaspoons (20 ml) passionflower tincture

4 teaspoons (20 ml) rose petal tincture

YIELD: 4 ounces (120 ml)

Combine all ingredients in a 4-ounce (120 ml) amber dropper bottle. Take 1 dropperful 3 times per day.

CALM VESSEL TEA

There are times I truly need a moment of calm, yet I just can't seem to slow down enough to get it. Drinking this tea helps a great deal in my efforts to get there.

1 ounce (28 g) dried oat straw

1 ounce (28 g) dried skullcap

½ ounce (14 g) dried chamomile flower

½ ounce (14 g) dried alfalfa

1 ounce (28 g) dried peppermint

YIELD: 4 ounces (112 g)

Combine all herbs; store in a glass jar. Make by the cup as needed: Steep 2 teaspoons (3 g) in 12 ounces (355 ml) of boiling water, covered, for 10 minutes.

PREGNANCY

Once you find yourself pregnant, your feelings can swing widely. Pregnancy can be emotionally and physically draining, but herbs can support you safely throughout. Stock your herbal home pantry with the following for pregnancy:

Alfalfa leaf

Ashwagandha root

Basil

Calendula flowers

Catnip

Chamomile flowers

Clove fruit

Comfrey leaf

Elderflowers

Fennel seed

Geranium leaves

Ginger root

Lavender flowers

Lemongrass

Nettle leaf

Orange peel

Peppermint

Red Raspberry leaf

Rose petals

Rosemary leaf

MORNING SICKNESS HERBAL ICE POPS

I find that ice pops seem to cut nausea off at the pass. Infuse the herbs and then freeze them for relief from morning (or anytime) sickness.

½ ounce (14 g) dried ginger root	YIELD: Varies depending on ice pop molds
½ ounce (14 g) dried lemongrass	Combine all ingredients in a saucepan. Pour
½ ounce (14 g) dried catnip leaf	3 quarts (3 liters) almost-boiling water over the
½ ounce (14 g) dried berries (raspberries, strawberries, or cranberries)	herbs and cover. Let steep for 1 hour. Strain and pour into ice pop molds; freeze. Enjoy as needed.

NAUSEA RELIEF TEA

Here's another delicious way to combat the ongoing struggle of nausea during pregnancy.

½ ounce (14 g) dried basil	YIELD: 3 ounces (84 g)
½ ounce (14 g) dried ginger	Combine all herbs; store in a glass jar. Make
2 ounces (56 g) dried peppermint	by the cup as needed: Steep 1 to 2 teaspoons (1.5 to 3 g) in 10 ounces (285 ml) of boiling water, covered, for 10 minutes.

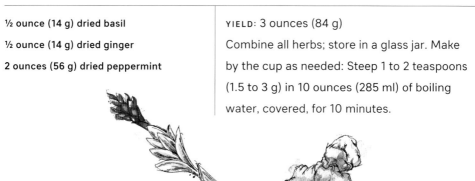

Ginger

YUCK MOUTH REFRESHER SPRAY

There is something about fresh breath that improves any situation. Use as needed for a little freshening up or at the onset of nausea to help temporarily reduce it.

1 ounce (28 ml) distilled water	YIELD: 1 ounce (28 ml)
10 drops peppermint and spearmint or cinnamon and clove essential oils	Pour water into a 1-ounce (28 ml) bottle with an atomizer; add essential oils and shake well.

MOM-TO-BE TEA

Maintaining our nutrient intake through tea is an excellent way to get B vitamins, calcium, and trace minerals. The tea is absorbed right through the digestive track and into the bloodstream to nourish ourselves and our baby and to tone the uterus as it grows and prepares for labor.

1 ounce (28 g) dried nettle leaf	YIELD: 3¼ ounces (91 g)
1 ounce (28 g) dried lemon balm leaf	Combine ingredients; store in a glass jar. Place
½ ounce (14 g) dried red raspberry leaf	3 tablespoons (13.5 g) of tea in 16 ounces (475 ml)
½ ounce (14 g) dried alfalfa leaf	hot water. Cover and let steep overnight; strain in
¼ ounce (7 g) dried ashwagandha root	the morning. Drink 1 to 2 cups per day for 10 to 12 weeks before due date.

PREGNANT BELLY OIL

Massaging your growing belly is an excellent way to connect with your baby. With the right combination of oils and herbs, you can also reduce stretch marks and overstretching of skin. Apply daily for best results. Some women love to slather it on; others prefer just enough to soak in to soften the skin. How much you use will determine how long it will last.

2 ounces (60 ml) coconut oil	YIELD: 8 ounces (235 ml)
2 ounces (60 ml) rosehip oil	Mix all ingredients together; store in an 8-ounce
2 ounces (60 ml) grapeseed oil	(235 ml) bottle. Label and keep in a cool,
2 ounces (60 ml) calendula oil	dark place.
40 drops frankincense essential oil	
20 drops orange essential oil	
10 drops ylang-ylang essential oil	

TUMMY TROUBLES TEA

Constipation is no stranger when changes in hormones are occurring. This gentle tea will help reduce bowel stagnation, reducing the promotion of hemorrhoids.

2 ounces (56 g) dried catnip leaf	**YIELD:** 4 ounces (112 g)
1 ounce (28 g) dried chamomile flowers	Combine all ingredients; store in a glass jar.
½ ounce (14 g) dried fennel seed	Steep 1 to 2 teaspoons (1.5 to 3 g) in 1 cup (235 ml)
½ ounce (14 g) dried ginger root	of boiling water, covered, for 8 to 10 minutes.
¼ ounce (7 g) dried cloves	

HERBAL SACHET FOR SLEEP

Some women sleep well during pregnancy; others struggle to get the rest they need. Having a sleep sachet next to the pillow can assist with relaxation and deeper sleep for some. Try mixing these or other herbs you like into the sachet; lay it next to or under your pillow while you sleep.

½ ounce (14 g) lavender flowers	**YIELD:** 1 sachet
½ ounce (14 g) rose petals	Combine all herbs and stuff them inside a cloth
¾ ounce (21 g) comfrey leaf	pouch. You can make a sachet pouch out of almost
¼ ounce (7 g) orange peel	any type of fabric. Cut two rectangles of fabric
⅛ ounce (3.5 g) geranium leaves	to the same size and pin them with right sides
	together. Stitch hems on three sides and then
	turn right side out. Fill the pouch with your herbal
	combination and stitch the remaining side closed.

HERBAL BATH FOR PREGNANCY

Extremely hot baths are not advised during pregnancy, but I think I would have been a hot mess without the ritual of my nightly relaxing bath. It gave me a moment to connect with the baby, myself, and what lay ahead.

2 ounces (56 g) dried rose petals	**YIELD:** 8 ounces (224 g)
2 ounces (56 g) dried lemongrass	Combine herbs; store in a glass jar until needed.
2 ounces (56 g) dried rosemary leaf	Put 6 to 8 tablespoons (27 to 36 g) in a muslin bag
2 ounces (56 g) dried jasmine flowers	and add to the bath as the water is running. Keep
	the bathroom door closed to keep the aromatic
	steam in the room.

PREGNANCY MASSAGE OIL

Having your partner or friend offer mini back, foot, or hand rubs can really make a difference in your pregnancy experience. Don't forget your partner during pregnancy! Offering to give your partner a little massage is a great way to say thank you for all his or her support.

1 ounce (28 g) dried rosemary leaf

½ ounce (14 g) dried chamomile flowers

½ ounce (14 g) dried rose petals

2 cups (475 ml) jojoba oil

40 drops rose essential oil

YIELD: 2 cups (475 ml)

Preheat oven to 170°F (77°C). Place herbs in a glass baking dish and pour enough jojoba oil over them to cover by 1 to 2 inches (3 to 5 cm). Bake for 4 hours. Allow to cool and then strain into a plastic squeeze bottle. Add rose essential oil.

PERINEUM STRETCH OIL

Many midwives recommend perineum massage daily during the last 6 to 8 weeks of pregnancy to help prepare for labor. Place one or two fingers on the opening of the lower vaginal canal and apply gentle pressure downward and then in a sweeping motion side to side in a U shape. This can help prepare the body for labor and is thought to reduce vaginal tearing.

¼ ounce (7 g) dried lavender flowers

¼ ounce (7 g) dried rose petals

¼ ounce (7 g) dried elder flowers

¼ ounce (7 g) dried comfrey leaf

1 cup (235 ml) grapeseed oil

60 drops rose essential oil

YIELD: 1 cup (235 ml)

Preheat oven to 170°F (77°C). Place herbs in a glass baking dish and pour enough grapeseed oil over them to cover by 1 to 2 inches (3 to 5 cm). Bake for 4 hours. Allow to cool; strain and store in a lidded container of your choice. Add rose essential oil and shake gently. Use enough oil to lubricate the fingers for an easy gliding motion.

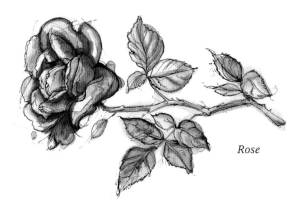

Rose

LABOR SUPPORT

I've had two children vaginally, and while I'd love to say I was one of those glorious goddesses who walked in the woods and sipped my herbal tea until I was ready to push, I was not. Labor rocked me. Beforehand, I prepared an entire labor kit to use for various things I might encounter. It included contraction regulators, pain supporters, herbs to encourage the cervix to ripen, an herbal soup packet to make and sip if my energy waned, and relaxation blends. I did get the chance to sip the soup, and I definitely utilized the pain tincture, but labor after my second pregnancy was so fast that most of it went by the wayside. Even so, I enjoyed being prepared and felt supported each day before the birth when I looked over my herbal allies.

Stock your home herbal pantry with the following for labor:

Ashwagandha root	Catnip leaf	Motherwort leaf
Astragalus root	Crampbark	Red Raspberry leaf
Black Cohosh	Fresh Ginger root	Schizandra berry
Blue Cohosh	Lycii berry	Skullcap leaf

TIP: Hydration is one of the key factors that can influence pain receptors during labor. Stay overhydrated during the last few weeks before birth. This super-hydration cushions the tissues surrounding the uterus and supports the uterus itself.

CONTRACTION INITIATION TEA

Only drink this tea if you are 40 weeks or more pregnant. Black cohosh is also helpful throughout labor if contractions stall.

3 tablespoons (72 g) black cohosh root **3 tablespoons (72 g) blue cohosh root**	YIELD: 2 pints (946 ml) Put blue cohosh in a pint jar (473 ml) and black cohosh in another pint jar. Fill both jars with hot water; allow them to steep for 4 hours or overnight. Strain and drink 6 ounces (175 ml), alternating jars, every 30 minutes for 4 hours. If you become nauseated, discontinue.

TEA TO ENCOURAGE THE OPENING OF THE CERVIX

When labor draws near, this tea can help open the cervix.

1- to 2-inch (3 to 5 cm) piece fresh ginger	YIELD: 1 cup tea
2 tablespoons (9 g) dried red raspberry leaf	Simmer fresh ginger in 1 quart (946 ml) of water. Turn off the heat and add 2 tablespoons (9 g) red raspberry leaf. Steep 1 to 2 hours. Drink 6 ounces (175 ml) every 20 minutes for 4 hours to encourage regular contractions and opening of the cervix once labor has begun.

LABOR PAIN SUPPORT TINCTURE

"Mind over matter," they say, but there was no way I could have meditated my way out of labor pain! This tincture allowed me a bit of reprieve and a moment to get my feet back on the ground.

1 tablespoon (15 ml) skullcap tincture	YIELD: 1 ounce (28 ml)
1 teaspoon (5 ml) catnip tincture	Combine all ingredients in a 1-ounce
1 teaspoon (5 ml) crampbark tincture	(28 ml) amber bottle with dropper. Take
1 teaspoon (5 ml) motherwort tincture	2 dropperfuls as needed throughout labor, typically every 60 minutes but can be every 1 to 2 hours.

HERBAL SOUP PACKET

Simmer the following herbs with vegetable or chicken stock for a nourishing and supportive broth to drink during labor.

1 whole astragalus root	YIELD: 32 ounces (946 ml) soup
½ ounce (14 ml) tincture schizandra berries	If you'd like to make this ahead of time,
½ ounce (14 ml) tincture lycii berries	combine the dried ingredients and store in
½ ounce (14 ml) tincture ashwagandha root	a glass jar in the pantry until ready to use.
32 ounces (946 ml) vegetable or chicken stock	Then, simply add to the stock and simmer for 1 to 2 hours, covered. Drink 8 ounces (235 ml) throughout labor to offer strength and nutrient support.

POSTPARTUM

Healing after labor can be as challenging as being a new mother. Luckily, our hormones are riding high, which eases the discomfort somewhat, but we still need to be cognizant of self-care during this time. Ask for assistance! As the new mother, no matter if this is your first child or your third, having support can create time for you to care for your body in its time of need. Having the following formulas on hand before labor is advisable.

Stock your home herbal pantry with the following for postpartum:

Anise seed	Fenugreek seed	Rosehips
Arnica flowers (fresh)	Goat's-Rue	Rosemary leaf
Astragalus root	Hop flowers	Schizandra berry
Basil leaf	Motherwort leaf	Skullcap
Beet powder	Nettle leaf	St. John's Wort
Blessed Thistle leaf	Nettle leaf	St. John's Wort (fresh)
Calendula flower	Oat Straw	Vitex berry
Comfrey leaf	Poplar buds (fresh)	Yellow Dock
Elderberry	Red Raspberry leaf	
Fennel seed	Rose petals	

POSTPARTUM SITZ BATH

Using herbs to heal the perineum and vaginal tearing will enable you to be more mobile and increase your overall comfort level. See page 243 for more on sitz baths.

1 ounce (28 g) comfrey leaf tincture

1 ounce (28 g) calendula flower tincture

1 ounce (28 g) basil leaf tincture

½ ounce (14 g) rose petal tincture

½ ounce (14 g) rosemary leaf tincture

YIELD: 4 ounces (112 g)

Combine all ingredients; store in a glass jar. Steep 5 tablespoons (22.5 g) in 1 quart (946 ml) of water for 2 to 4 hours or overnight. Strain the herbs out and save them for a second infusing if desired. Warm the infusion and add to sitz bath basin. Add 1 to 2 quarts (946 to 1892 ml) warm water if desired and submerge the perineum twice daily, if possible, for 7 to 10 days.

HERBAL BLOOD BUILDING SYRUP

If excessive blood loss occurred during labor, your stores need to be replenished.
The herbs in this formula are traditionally used for blood building and iron fortifying.

½ ounce (14 g) dried yellow dock	YIELD: 4 cups (940 ml)
½ ounce (14 g) dried rosehips	Gently simmer herbs in 4 cups (950 ml)
½ ounce (14 g) dried beet powder	water over medium-low heat until water
¼ ounce (7 g) dried anise seed	is reduced by half. Strain, add honey,
¼ ounce (7 g) dried elderberry	and stir until completely dissolved. Take
1 to 2 cups (340 to 680 g) honey	2 teaspoons (10 ml) twice daily.

POST-DELIVERY RECOVERY TINCTURE FOR STAMINA

Labor is exhausting. Having a newborn is exhausting. This blend helps gently support you
without stimulating your baby, if you're breastfeeding.

2 tablespoons (30 ml) astragalus root tincture	YIELD: 4 ounces (120 ml)
2 tablespoons (30 ml) schizandra berry tincture	Combine all extracts in a 4-ounce (120 ml)
1 tablespoon (15 ml) nettle leaf tincture	amber dropper bottle. Take 1 dropperful
1 tablespoon (15 ml) calendula flower tincture	2 or 3 times per day.
1 tablespoon (15 ml) elderberry tincture	
1 tablespoon (15 ml) comfrey leaf tincture	

MOTHER'S FLOW TEA

Relax, stay calm, and try this formula to support breast milk production.

1 ounce (28 g) dried goat's-rue	YIELD: 4 ounces (112 g)
1 ounce (28 g) dried fennel seed	Combine all ingredients; store in a glass
1 ounce (28 g) dried fenugreek seed	jar. Make medicinal strength (see page
½ ounce (14 g) dried nettle leaf	245). Drink 3 cups daily for 8 to 12 weeks.
½ ounce (14 g) dried red raspberry leaf	
½ ounce (14 g) dried blessed thistle leaf	
⅛ ounce (3.5 g) dried hop flowers	

MOTHER'S FLOW TINCTURE

If you'd prefer your breast milk production assistance in tincture form, this recipe is for you.

2 tablespoons (30 ml) goat's-rue tincture	YIELD: 4 ounces (120 ml)
4 teaspoons (20 ml) fennel seed tincture	Combine all ingredients in a 4-ounce
4 teaspoons (20 ml) fenugreek seed tincture	(120 ml) amber dropper bottle. Take
4 teaspoons (20 ml) blessed thistle leaf tincture	2 dropperfuls 3 times per day.
2 teaspoons (10 ml) nettle leaf tincture	
2 teaspoons (10 ml) red raspberry leaf tincture	
2 teaspoons (10 ml) hop flower tincture	

C-SECTION TOPICAL TREATMENT

Caesarians are tough to heal from. This treatment aims to reduce swelling and tenderness.

1 ounce (28 ml) poplar oil	YIELD: 4 ounces (120 ml)
1 ounce (28 ml) arnica oil	Combine the first four oils in a 4-ounce
1 ounce (28 ml) St. John's wort oil	(120 ml) bottle and then add the rose
1 ounce (28 ml) comfrey leaf oil	essential oil. Shake gently to combine.
25 drops rose essential oil	Apply 3 times per day around the incisions.

POSTPARTUM DEPRESSION TINCTURE

The rise and fall of hormones throughout and after pregnancy can greatly affect the mother's personality. I often see women who believe they are incapable of bonding with their baby, yet after using hormone-balancing herbs and treatments, they realize the chemical imbalance in their body, not their lack of love, was to blame. Herbs may not always help postpartum depression, but they are a good place to begin.

1 tablespoon (15 ml) motherwort leaf tincture	YIELD: 2 ounces (60 ml)
1 tablespoon (15 ml) vitex berry tincture	Combine all ingredients in a 2-ounce (60 ml)
2 teaspoons (10 ml) St. John's wort tincture	amber dropper bottle. Take 1 dropperful
2 teaspoons (10 ml) skullcap tincture	3 times per day for 1 to 2 months. If symp-
2 teaspoons (10 ml) oat straw tincture	toms worsen or do not diminish, please
	consult your natural health care provider.

Throughout the Living years, may you be blessed with health, happiness, and prosperity. Use your strength to take you beyond your dreams and use herbs to support you along the journey.

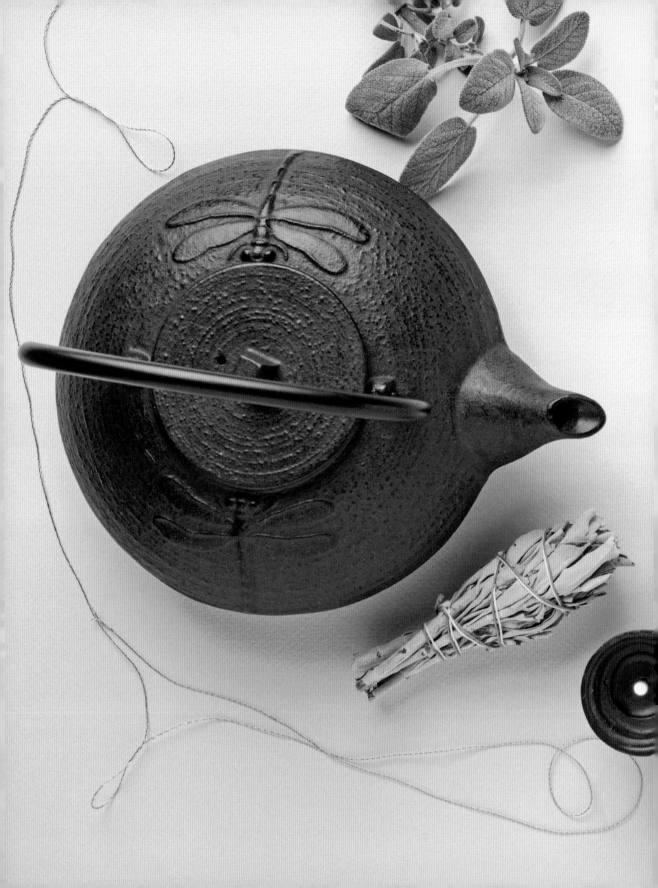

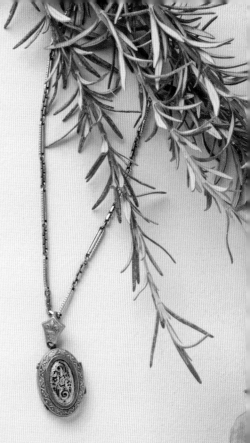

CHAPTER 5

Fulfillment

Menopause and Beyond

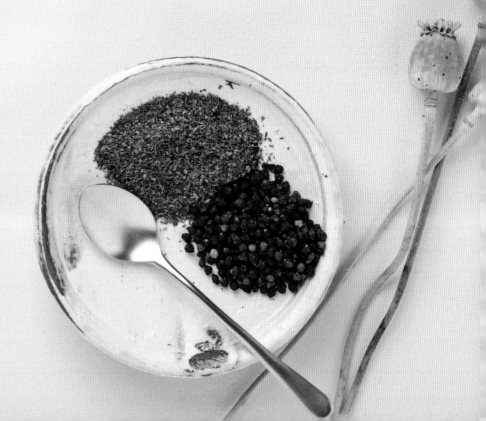

AS I ATTEMPT TO MOVE THROUGH MY FORTIES as gracefully as I can, life never ceases teach me new lessons—or the same old ones over and over. As someone who thrives on personal growth, I welcome these opportunities to learn more about how I walk through the world communicating with myself and engaging others. Sometimes, the lessons are gentle nudges of remembrance; other times, it's as though I've just been run over by a bus. Our physical and emotional experiences shape us as we move through life. They can better us, break us, or sometimes go completely unnoticed. But each time we do notice them, it's an opportunity to gain another piece of understanding, another piece to fill our basket with fulfillment. I truly used to think that by the time I reached middle age, which begins at age forty-five, I would be at peace with my life and myself. It goes to prove that we never stop learning if we continue to seek out new opportunities and ways in which to grow.

When I was a young herbalist, I was always interested in the female body and the herbs to support it. Perhaps my own body inspired me, as I was often fascinated by everything it could do and how easily it was influenced. I took several concentrated courses in women's health, allowing me to gain valuable and applicable knowledge. One of the nice things about studying health, and herbal medicine in particular, is its ability to be applied readily. You can find a tea section in almost any grocery store and begin using herbs today if you'd like. That accessibility is immensely valuable to our communities and important for personalized health care.

One area of women's health that I've always been drawn to is menopause. Although our society seems to begin seriously discounting woman as valuable after the age of fifty, I have always found this time in a women's life to be filled with intention and purpose. Women over fifty tend to have a sense of resolve with themselves and the world around them. They all speak of having a stronger sense of self-confidence and an easier time navigating strife and struggle should it come up in their lives. Naturally, experience plays a part in this, but I'm keen to believe it runs deeper than that. After fifty years of living, I think we all deserve to have respect and peace in our lives. The only way to guarantee that is from within; we can't always control our finances, health, relationships, jobs, and other external influences. But as we get older, we can look to ourselves to find inner fulfillment. Many years ago, while traveling, I found myself in a poverty-stricken country that offered its citizens little hope of escape. Despite this, I continuously came across older women whose smiles repeatedly met mine. They had little in the way of material wealth, but they spoke to me about how happy and fulfilled they were in their lives. They had family and music, and they were grateful every day. I will never forget how bright their eyes shone when we spoke. It was a clear message that the true path to health and fulfillment began with inner happiness.

The first parts of our lives are extremely outward focused. Going to school, working, and perhaps having children all require an extreme amount of outward energy. Both menstruation and pregnancy are physical and energetic releases out of the body. For thirty-some years, most women menstruate and ride the hormone highway each month. They also pursue education, manifest careers, raise children, support families, and attempt to balance the persistent voices from our media and society telling us we need to do more. Meanwhile, their equal rights, pay, and progression are suppressed. All this needs to be considered when we speak of health and wellness, as it can directly correlate to the state of our well-being.

When we reach perimenopause/menopause, the energy that was once used to conduct the ebb and flow of menstruation ceases. The hormones that have been going up and down for years and years readjust to the new normal of no menstruation. Consider the emotional impact this amazing shift has on women. Some grieving is normal—the grieving for a time past, for birthing no more children, and perhaps fear of the future. Ultimately, the understanding of what it means to radically shift our hormones is of utmost importance and needs to be evaluated.

Hormones in general can affect our mood, our decisions, and how we view the outside world and ourselves. For some, the years of menstruation are a perpetual balance of understanding what is a hormonal response and what is a true interpersonal one. Even though they may all be the latter, hormones can accentuate our truest feelings. When the hormones begin to diminish due to absence of ovulation and menstruation, yet another emotional shift can occur as well. Our body is now utilizing the extra energy in other areas of our body for health and healing, and the lack of hormones, which can cause symptomatic complaints (more on that in a minute), often catapults us into a new emotional paradigm.

As you might guess, the initial drop in hormones can be uncomfortable. Some of my patients report feeling extremely irritable or crazy. When we tease out these statements, it's obvious that they are not acting like this outright, but that it is more of a constant internal feeling of discomfort. I think we can only expect this to be normal. Your hormones are no longer acting as they have for the past thirty years of your life; your internal systems are shifting, and that's going to feel quite different. Give the process time, and herbal support, to ease the transition and lessen the possible symptoms of your body's new way of operating. As herbalist and medical consultant Amanda McQuade Crawford once said, "Changes that accompany menopause are no less dramatic than those we experienced at puberty."

So that we are all on the same page, let's talk about menopause. Menopause occurs when the ovaries stop releasing eggs and menstruation ceases. "Pre-menopause" can begin eight to ten years before complete menopause and occurs when the normal monthly cycle of ovulation and menstruation becomes less regular. This entire period of transition is also known as the "climacteric" phase, because the reproductive phase of life is reaching its climax. The widely used term is *perimenopause*, meaning "the time surrounding menopausal changes."

Pre-menopause is usually a gradual process, so women may not know exactly when it begins. If women are reasonably healthy and older than thirty-six, an irregular cycle may be a sign of pre-menopause. Pre-menopause commonly begins in the forties, but it can start earlier for various reasons. Genetics, high-stress lifestyles, emotional issues, socioeconomic influences, environmental concerns, and gynecological problems may contribute to early onset of pre-menopause. I recommended talking to your female relatives about cycle patterns as a means to gauge your own. With all our modern influences, things seem to be shifting, but such discussions can still provide helpful information.

Signs and symptoms of menopause include hot flashes, night sweats, insomnia, vaginal dryness, vaginal thinning, vaginal irritation, an inability to climax, decreased libido, and emotional shifts. But at least eight of these nine symptoms can also be caused by other things. Always see your health practitioner of choice to talk through any shift you are experiencing. This can help determine causes you might not have considered. I had a younger patient who was convinced she was beginning perimenopause because she was suddenly experiencing intense night sweats. After a thorough conversation proving perimenopause was unlikely, I asked her about her bedding. She was someone who typically ran cold and had a lot of blankets on her bed. Considering this, and that we had just changed seasons from winter to spring, I asked her to remove one of the blankets from the bed. She e-mailed three days later to report that the night sweats were gone. I'm not downplaying physical symptoms; my point is that discussing your symptoms with someone can sometimes result in simple solutions.

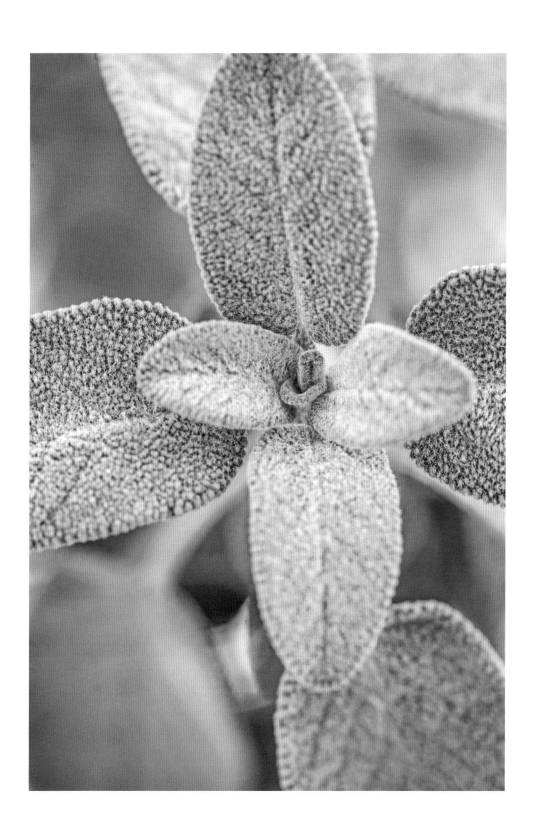

A SHIFT IN THE VAGINA

Two of the most common complaints of perimenopause and menopause are vaginal thinning and dryness. These are most often due to declining estrogen levels. The effects of decreasing estrogen happen over time and vary from woman to woman. Thinning, irritation, and dryness are the results, as well as the labia being reabsorbed over time. Estrogen helps keep the vaginal tissues fat and plump, and with their levels declining, the vagina actually redesigns itself. The labia minora may eventually disappear, and the vaginal canal gets smaller. The vaginal walls become thinner, and the vaginal tissue becomes less cornified, meaning durable and tough. The vaginal canal of a younger woman is all cornified for intercourse purposes. This typically protects the vagina from penetration and friction. When the cornification of the tissue transitions, vaginal tissue can easily be irritated during sex and at times may bleed afterward. During perimenopause and menopause, hormonal imbalance may thin or dry the lining of the vagina, causing it to become inflamed or sensitive. If a woman is experiencing discomfort during sex or the vaginal dryness persists despite normal sexual desire, it may indicate atrophic vaginitis—the term used for chronic vaginal inflammation.

Another anatomical result of decreased estrogen is that the cervix can become shallower, and its size typically decreases.

When a woman has not had a menstrual cycle for twelve consecutive months, she is considered menopausal. The time before that is the perimenopause phase. This is when ovulation and menses become irregular and hormones are attempting to reregulate. Conception is still possible, but the viability of the eggs greatly decreases during this time. As any woman in her forties can tell you, the days of increased vaginal moisture during sex have slowly disappeared. Decreased estrogen leads to the vaginal glands secreting less mucus, which can make sex irritating to the vaginal canal unless lubrication is used or additional foreplay brings about natural lubrication. The woman's body is fascinating. Although our ability to conceive diminishes and the body reorients itself, the changes aren't all bad. Read the "Libido" section below to learn how our body's reproduction focus turns into pleasure focus during the Fulfillment phase.

Herbs have been used for centuries to liberate the stored estrogen of the body. Throughout our lives, certain hormones are metabolized into estrogen for storage in our fat cells. This is yet another way in which the body amazes me. This storage is saved for the Fulfillment phase. The body knows, understands, and prepares for the need of estrogen later in life by storing small amounts in fats cells to be utilized as we enter menopause. It is a lifelong preparation. Once we enter menopause and estrogen production drops, we liberate estrogen from fat cells. It enters the bloodstream and can be utilized.

There are two approaches to using herbs during the Fulfillment phase. One is to support what hormones we already have available to us versus introducing new exogenous forms of hormone replacement. By freeing the stored estrogen from fat, you are giving your body the small increments it needs to maintain physiological balance. Herbs that support the liver can help reduce undesirable symptoms. Herbs that promote progesterone production are valuable for maintaining the balance of the reproductive hormones; this in turn can keep vaginal tissues healthy, reduce vaginal irritation, balance the pH of the vagina, and possibly improve libido. Herbs are also used to reduce or clear the body of the symptoms that can accompany menopause.

Another approach is to use herbs that demonstrate estrogen effects; they're called estrogenic herbs. To determine if you want to use them, you must understand how these herbs work in the body. Estrogenic herbs are classified as such when they have a high percentage of isoflavones present. Isoflavones, which fall under the flavonoid grouping, can mimic estrogen in the body. When we enter the Fulfillment part of our lives, estrogen is greatly diminished. This dip in estrogen can contribute to menopausal symptoms such as hot flashes, insomnia, vaginal changes, and bone loss. Using estrogenic or phytoestrogen herbs can offer the body micro amounts of estrogen-like substances to reduce the symptoms. Foods containing phytoestrogens include beans, soy products, peas, lentils, and whole grains and seeds, especially flaxseed, rye, and millet. Herbs that contain phytoestrogens include red clover, alfalfa, hops, licorice, thyme, and lemon verbena. Some herbs that mimic phytoestrogens but do not have their true characteristics are black cohosh, dong quai, and ginseng. Research is regularly conducted with phytoestrogens; although concrete stances have not been determined, it is generally believed that phytoestrogens work much differently than naturally produced estrogen in the body. They aren't considered to lead to estrogen dominance or excess estrogen production. They tend to have selective qualities on receptive sites, working to create balance in the body. We honestly cannot yet say if phytoestrogen herbs should or should not be used if you have an estrogen-driven cancer. One thing we do know is that the abundance of xenoestrogens—chemicals that surround us that mimic estrogen in the body—are a leading cause of hormone disruption and gene expression, leading to disease and chronic pathologies.

When evaluating how to care for the vagina as we enter the Fulfillment part of our life, we must consider stress. Stress at this point in our lives can directly affect the health of the vagina and our libido. It has a way of perpetuating habits that may feel good in the moment but have detrimental effects. These can include excessive sugar, fat, or caffeine intake and a lack of proper hydration. Stress can perpetuate the need to complete one more task in order to feel that it's safe to relax. Or it can result in a habit of putting everyone else's needs before your own. Finding regular moments for yourself is vital at this time of your life. Balancing the physical transitions with inner calm can produce powerful shifts toward peace in your daily life.

Reminder: Being and identifying as a woman who possesses a uterus is a blessing, not a curse. If you feel you've been moving from one aspect of your life to another with nothing but negative uterine experiences, I wish something better for you. Suffering through menstruation and perhaps reproduction only to move into five to ten years of miserable menopausal symptoms is not a way to live. Let the herbs help. Seek out a new care provider to help you achieve a higher quality of life. You are worth it, and you have too much to offer this world to be sidelined due to hormonal imbalance.

Common Physical Complaints of the Fulfillment Phase

Vagina health	Mineral nourishment and	Brain support
Libido	osteoporosis	Thinning hair
Hormone regulation	Sleep and stress support	Prolapse

VAGINAL HEALTH

Caring for every part of our body, including our vagina, is important as we age. Caring for the delicate tissues and ensuring proper flora allow us to be comfortable in our body.

Stock your home herbal pantry with the following for vaginal health:

Calendula flower	Comfrey leaves
Chamomile flower	Elderflowers

VAGINAL DRYNESS ESSENTIAL OIL BLEND

Apply twice daily to external vaginal tissue and tissue at introitus. You can use this blend anytime to soothe irritation.

1½ tablespoons (25 ml) jojoba oil

1 teaspoon (5 ml) vitamin E oil

25 drops helichrysum essential oil

15 drops ylang-ylang essential oil

YIELD: 1 ounce (28 ml)

Combine all ingredients in a 1-ounce (28 ml) bottle. Gently mix.

VAGINAL TISSUE HEALER SALVE

When irritation or bleeding occurs, apply this gentle tissue healer 3 times per day.

½ ounce (14 g) dried chamomile flower

½ ounce (14 g) dried calendula flower

½ ounce (14 g) dried comfrey leaves

½ ounce (14 g) dried elderflowers

1 cup (235 ml) olive oil

1 teaspoon (5 ml) vitamin E oil

1 ounce (28 g) beeswax

60 drops rose essential oil

YIELD: 8 ounces (224 g)

Preheat oven to 170°F (77°C). Place herbs in a glass baking dish and cover with olive oil. Bake for 4 hours. Strain. Add the vitamin E oil and then transfer to a saucepan. Heat over low heat while adding the beeswax; stir until completely melted. Remove from the heat and add rose essential oil; pour into container of choice.

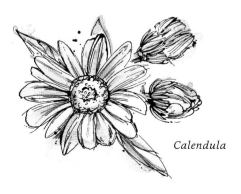

Calendula

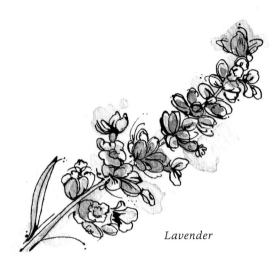

Lavender

HERBAL LUBRICATION

This can be used anytime to soothe dry tissues, but it is also safe to use during sex to lubricate the vagina. There are plenty of essential oils to choose from: Lavender is relaxing, jasmine and ylang-ylang are aphrodisiacs, rose and helichrysum are healing for skin tissues, and peppermint and rosemary give a little spice should you so desire.

1 ounce (28 g) dried comfrey leaf

1 cup (218 g) coconut oil

2 teaspoons (10 ml) aloe vera gel

Essential oils such as lavender, peppermint, rosemary, jasmine, rose, ylang-ylang, or helichrysum (optional)

YIELD: 1 cup (235 ml)

Preheat oven to 170°F (77°C). Place comfrey in a glass baking dish and pour enough coconut oil over it to cover by 1 to 2 inches (3 to 5 cm). Bake for 4 hours. Allow to cool and then strain into a bowl. Add aloe vera gel; mix well. At this point you can add essential oils if you'd like; I'd keep it to around 40 to 60 drops your first round. You can always adjust to your preference with your second batch.

LIBIDO

Throughout my years studying menopause, one subject has continually fascinated me: the better orgasm. All we ever hear about in the media is that menopausal women have no sex drive or ability to climax. Well, my studies show differently. Although sexual interest might take some more inspiration, the menopausal vagina is primed and poised for great things. The thinning of the vaginal walls actually accesses nerve endings in a new way, making them more easily excitable. The lack of immediate moisture demands that purposeful and sensual touch be used to elicit excitement. This takes time and allows the body to respond in a slower, but ultimately stronger way. I encourage all my patients, women and men, to utilize this information to engage in new ways to stimulate each other; both will reap the rewards.

Stock your home herbal pantry with the following for libido:

Ashwagandha root

Cardamom

Cinnamon

Damiana leaf

Ginger

Licorice root

Maca root

Nutmeg

Passionflower leaf

Rose petals

Shatavari root

Tribulus

Vanilla bean

Passionflower

LIBIDO TONIC TEA

As hormones change, so does libido. Using herbs such as maca and tribulus has been known for centuries to improve sex drive by balancing hormones.

1½ ounces (42 g) shatavari root	YIELD: 4 ounces (112 g)
1 ounce (28 g) maca root	Combine all ingredients; store in a
1 ounce (28 g) tribulus	glass jar. Make medicinal strength
¼ ounce (7 g) licorice root	(see page 245), and drink 2 cups daily
¼ ounce (7 g) rose petals	for 6 to 8 weeks.

IN THE MOOD TINCTURE

When you wish to set the mood, take this an hour beforehand and find that special someone to get close to.

2 teaspoons (10 ml) passionflower leaf tincture	YIELD: 1 ounce (28 ml)
1 teaspoon (5 ml) damiana leaf tincture	Combine all extracts in a 1-ounce
1 teaspoon (5 ml) licorice root tincture	(28 ml) amber dropper bottle.
1 teaspoon (5 ml) ashwagandha root tincture	Take 1 to 2 dropperfuls as needed.
1 teaspoon (5 ml) California poppy flower tincture	

APHRODISIAC ESSENTIAL OIL BLEND

This is a great blend to add to a diffuser in the bedroom. It focuses on relaxation and stimulation of the excitement centers.

1 teaspoon (5 ml) ylang-ylang oil	YIELD: 2 teaspoons (10 ml)
½ teaspoon (2.5 ml) rosewood oil	Combine all oils in a 10 ml essential oil bottle.
½ teaspoon (2.5 ml) cardamom oil	Use 5 drops in a room diffuser as desired.

HERBAL APHRODISIAC CHOCOLATE

Many of our culinary spices have healing potential. Here's one way to spice up more than the kitchen.

1 cup (218 g) cocoa butter	YIELD: 12 balls
¾ cup (255 g) honey	In a double boiler, slowly heat cocoa
1 cup (86 g) raw cacao powder	butter over very low heat until melted.
1 teaspoon (5 ml) vanilla extract	Slowly stir in honey until completely
1 teaspoon (2.3 g) ground cinnamon	mixed. Stir in the remaining ingredients
⅛ teaspoon ground nutmeg	and pour into molds. Chill in the refrigerator
¼ teaspoon ground ginger	for up to 4 weeks. Share 1 to 2 with a lover.
¼ teaspoon ground cardamom	
½ teaspoon vanilla bean powder	
Pinch of sea salt	

HORMONE REGULATION

When our hormones are transitioning to the menopausal state, they need support to reestablish a new normal. This is a great time for herbal hormonal tonics. These formulas should be used for 8 to 12 weeks to gently work with the body in establishing healthy balance.

Stock your home herbal pantry with the following for hormone regulation:

Black Cohosh

Dong Quai

Eleuthero root

Lemon Balm leaf

Licorice root

Maca root

Nettle leaf

Partridgeberry

Rhodiola root bark

Sage leaf

Spirulina powder

Tribulus

Vitex berry

Yellow Dock root

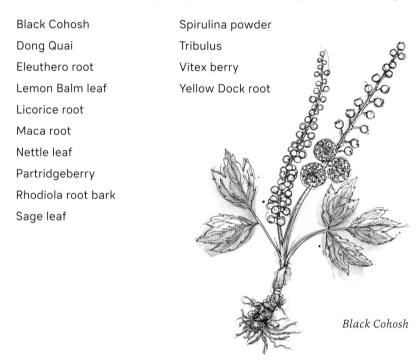

Black Cohosh

HORMONE BALANCE TINCTURE

Resetting the hormone balance may take time, but this formula is known to help.

2 teaspoons (10 ml) maca tincture	**YIELD:** 1 ounce (28 ml)
2 teaspoons (10 ml) tribulus tincture	Combine all extracts in a 1-ounce (28 ml)
1 teaspoon (5 ml) dong quai tincture	amber dropper bottle. Take 1 dropperful
½ teaspoon (2.5 ml) nettle leaf tincture	3 times per day.
½ teaspoon (2.5 ml) sage leaf tincture	

HORMONE BALANCE THROUGH THE LIVER

This tincture will help balance your hormones via supporting the liver.

2 teaspoons (10 ml) yellow dock root tincture	**YIELD**: 1 ounce (28 ml)
1 teaspoon (5 ml) partridgeberry tincture	Combine all extracts in a 1-ounce (28 ml)
1 teaspoon (5 ml) black cohosh tincture	amber dropper bottle. Take 1 dropperful
1 teaspoon (5 ml) licorice root tincture	3 times per day.
1 teaspoon (5 ml) vitex berry tincture	

ENDOCRINE SUPPORT CAPSULES

This formula is geared toward supporting the overall endocrine system. A vital blend to support every system, it can be used like a daily endocrine herbal vitamin.

½ ounce (14 g) spirulina powder	**YIELD**: 200 capsules
½ ounce (14 g) eleuthero root powder	Mix all ingredients in a bowl. Use the
½ ounce (14 g) lemon balm leaf powder	mixture to fill empty vegetable capsules.
¼ ounce (7 g) vitex berry powder	Take 2 capsules once or twice daily.
¼ ounce (7 g) rhodiola root bark powder	

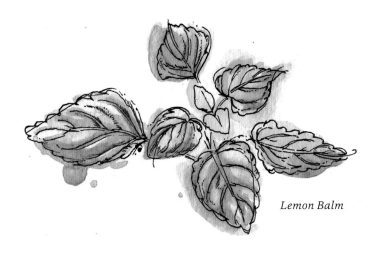

Lemon Balm

BONE HEALTH

As we age, our bones need careful consideration. When we have a decreased output of estrogen, we lose the production of bone osteoblast cells, which stimulate bone growth. As a result, osteoclasts, the cells that absorb bone, end up absorbing more bone than we make. This is why bone-strengthening exercise is so highly valued in later years. You strengthen the bone and also liberate estrogen to support bone growth. Calcium deficiency is also a problem. I wish we could eat our way to calcium balance, but that seems to be proving harder as years go by and our soils become more and more depleted. Although supplemental calcium is helpful, it can be hard to extract from vitamins, making deficiency common. Drinking high calcium teas and herbs that support the hormonal aspect of bone growth are one positive thing you can do.

Stock your home herbal pantry with the following for osteoporosis:

Alfalfa leaf	Dandelion leaf	Peppermint leaf
Black Cohosh root	Green tea	Rosehip powder
Chickweed leaf powder	Hawthorn berry	St. John's Wort
	Horsetail leaf	Yellow Dock root powder
Comfrey leaf	Nettle leaf	

OSTEOPOROSIS FIGHTING TEA

This is a daily tonic tea to support the bones through herbal mineralization.

½ ounce (14 g) dried nettle leaf	YIELD: 4 ounces (112 g)
½ ounce (14 g) dried alfalfa leaf	Combine all ingredients; store in a
½ ounce (14 g) dried comfrey leaf	glass jar. Make medicinal strength
½ ounce (14 g) dried horsetail leaf	(see page 245), and drink 2 cups daily
2 ounces (56 g) peppermint leaf	for 8 to 12 weeks.

OSTEOPOROSIS TINCTURE BLEND

This daily tonic tincture supports the bones through herbal mineralization.

2 teaspoons (10 ml) hawthorn berry tincture	YIELD: 1 ounce (28 ml)
1 teaspoon (5 ml) black cohosh root tincture	Combine all extracts in a 1-ounce (28 ml)
1 teaspoon (5 ml) St. John's wort tincture	amber dropper bottle. Take 1 dropperful
1 teaspoon (5 ml) nettle leaf tincture	3 times per day for 4 to 6 months.
1 teaspoon (5 ml) alfalfa leaf tincture	

APPLE CIDER VINEGAR OSTEOPOROSIS BLEND

I also recommend making your own herbal vinegars. I used them as salad dressings, or they can be taken the same as the tincture. Using herbal medicine as food is a great way to support the body.

Ingredients	Instructions
2 tablespoons (9 g) dried hawthorn berry 2 tablespoons (9 g) dried black cohosh root 1 tablespoon (4.5 g) dried St. John's wort 1 tablespoon (4.5 g) dried nettle leaf 1 tablespoon (4.5 g) dried alfalfa leaf Apple cider vinegar	YIELD: 1 pint Put herbs in a pint jar; fill to the top with apple cider vinegar. Close tightly and give it a good shake. Store in a cool dark cupboard for 4 weeks, remembering to shake it every day. Strain the mixture after 4 weeks; use daily.

MINERAL CAPSULES

Trace minerals offer a lot to the body in terms of healing and support. They work on the function and structure of the body in many ways vitamins cannot.

Ingredients	Instructions
½ ounce (14 g) alfalfa leaf powder ½ ounce (14 g) yellow dock root powder ¼ ounce (7 g) dandelion leaf powder ¼ ounce (7 g) nettle leaf powder ¼ ounce (7 g) chickweed leaf powder ¼ ounce (7 g) rosehip powder	YIELD: 200 capsules Combine all ingredients in a bowl. Use the mixture to fill empty vegetable capsules. Take 2 capsules once or twice daily as a supplement.

Green Tea

Research shows that drinking green tea regularly has positive results in reducing bone density loss. It also shows the reduction in elderly bone fractures in those who drank green tea regularly. Regularly, by the way, would be 5 to 8 cups per week.

HOT FLASHES

Hot flashes are the body's natural way to control internal temperature. They release internal heat through the skin in an attempt to cool the body off. When they occur at night, they are called night sweats. Unfortunately, we still haven't nailed down what causes the rise in body temperature that makes the hypothalamus stimulate the brain to release heat in this way, but it is thought to have something to do with the drop in estrogen. Using the hormone balancing recipes listed on pages 165 to 168 may be the ticket to correcting the imbalance, but you can use the following to address the symptoms.

Stock your home herbal pantry with the following for hot flashes:

Black Cohosh	Gingko leaf	Rosemary
Borage leaf	Hibiscus	Sage leaf
Bupleurum root	Lavender flowers	Shatavari root
Burdock root	Linden leaf and flower	Wild Yam
Chamomile flowers	Maca root	Yarrow flowers
Chickweed	Marshmallow root	
Cleavers	Peppermint leaf	

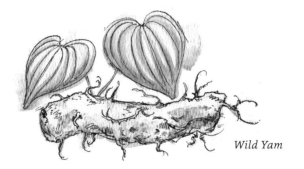

Wild Yam

HOT FLASH TINCTURE

When hot flashes arise, consider using this tonic to shift the patterns, cool down, and redistribute the heat.

2½ teaspoons (10 ml) black cohosh tincture

2 teaspoons (10 ml) sage leaf tincture

¾ teaspoon (4 ml) maca root tincture

½ teaspoon (2 ml) gingko leaf tincture

½ teaspoon (2 ml) shatavari root tincture

YIELD: 1 ounce (28 ml)

Combine all extracts in a 1-ounce (28 ml) amber dropper bottle. Take 1 dropperful 3 times per day.

HOT FLASH ACUTE TEA

This blend is for when you are suffering from acute hot flashes. Take as needed to find temporary relief.

1 ounce (28 g) dried sage leaf	YIELD: 4 ounces (112 g)
1 ounce (28 g) dried black cohosh	Combine all herbs and store in a glass jar.
2 ounces (56 g) dried peppermint leaf	Make tea by the cup as needed: Place 2 teaspoons (3 g) of tea in 12 ounces (355 ml) water; simmer, covered, over medium heat for 10 minutes. Turn off the heat and add another ½ teaspoon (1 g) tea; cover and let steep for 5 minutes. Or make medicinal strength (see page 245) to have on hand and drink as needed.

HOT FLASH ACUTE TINCTURE

An alternative to tea, this tincture will also help you when you're having a hot flash.

1½ teaspoons (8 ml) sage leaf tincture	YIELD: 1 ounce (28 ml)
1½ teaspoons (8 ml) bupleurum root tincture	Combine all ingredients in a 2-ounce (60 ml) amber dropper bottle. Take 1 dropperful 3 times per day as a preventative or take as needed to reduce acute symptoms.
¾ teaspoon (4 ml) wild yam tincture	
¾ teaspoon (4 ml) black cohosh tincture	
1¼ teaspoons (4 ml) peppermint tincture	

TEA FOR KEEPING IT COOL

Here is another tea option for the summer. Hot flashes or not, this is a great blend to cool down quickly.

1 ounce (28 g) dried hibiscus	YIELD: 4 ounces (112 g)
1 ounce (28 g) dried marshmallow root	Combine all herbs and store in a glass jar.
1 ounce (28 g) dried chamomile flowers	Make tea by the cup as needed: Steep
½ ounce (14 g) dried linden leaf and flower	2 teaspoons (3 g) in 12 ounces (355 ml)
½ ounce (14 g) dried borage leaf	of water, covered, for 10 minutes.

COOLING BATH

Sometimes a bath is just what the doctor ordered for a good night's sleep.

Ingredients	Instructions
1 ounce (28 g) dried sage **½ ounce (14 g) dried rosemary** **½ ounce (14 g) dried lavender** **½ ounce (14 g) dried yarrow flowers**	YIELD: 1 bath Fill a large muslin bag with herbs and add it to your bath.

CASTOR OIL FOR HOT FLASHES

On an intuitive hit, I recommended the following castor oil pack to a patient suffering from night sweats. She wasn't ready to take anything internally but was seeking suggestions. One of castor oil's greatest gifts is support of the liver. Considering the liver's relationship to hormones, I thought we'd give it a try. After using it one time, she found relief. In cases like this, I document the success and begin incorporating it with other patients. It has proven its value repeatedly.

½ ounce (14 g) dried chickweed

½ ounce (14 g) dried cleavers

½ ounce (14 g) dried burdock root

½ ounce (14 g) dried sage leaf

Castor oil

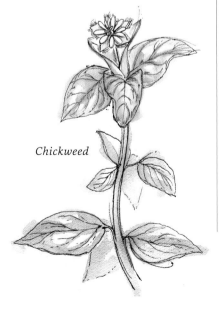

Chickweed

YIELD: 2 cups (475 ml)

Preheat oven to 170°F (77°C). Place herbs in a glass baking dish and pour enough castor oil over them to cover by 1 to 2 inches (3 to 5 cm). Bake for 4 hours. Allow to cool and then strain the mixture into a storage container. Apply 1 to 2 tablespoons (15 to 30 ml) over your entire abdomen. You don't need to rub it in. Place a cotton flannel over your abdomen and apply gentle heat from a heating pad or hot water bottle. Relax and rest for 30 minutes. Or go to bed and simply throw the flannel or hot water bottle on the floor at some point during the night.

Note: Be sure your bedding is weather appropriate. I love a down comforter as much as the next gal, but ensure that it's not making you too hot, exacerbating your night sweats.

SLEEP AND STRESS

Once again, we return to the adrenals when considering menopause symptoms. In reviewing our adrenal health, we need to ask ourselves how much stress we carry day to day. And if we do have a certain amount of stress, how is it manifesting in our body? In our relationships? What physical complaints are we experiencing, and which of them could be attributed to adrenal insufficiency? My patients are often surprised at the list of complaints that is revealed, as they've suppressed the acknowledgment of the symptom for so long. They've simply learned to live with it. Stress takes many forms, both physical and emotional, and treating it will bring a sense of well-being back faster than almost anything I've seen. Refer to chapter 7 for guidance on supporting the stress centers of the body: the adrenal glands and the central nervous system.

Stock your home herbal pantry with the following for sleep and stress:

Angelica root	Hops	Turmeric root
Chamomile flower	Lemon Balm	Wild Yam root
Chickweed	Sage leaf	Wood Betony
Eleuthero root	Skullcap	
Hawthorn leaf and	Spirulina	
flower	St. John's Wort	

Mediation

I won't claim to be a regular meditator, but research has repeatedly shown the advantages of meditation and stress reduction.

CENTERING TEA

This tea is recommended for moments when you need to calm and center yourself. Taking 10 minutes to make and drink a cup of tea can reframe your day.

1 ounce (28 g) dried lemon balm	YIELD: 2 ounces (56 g)
½ ounce (14 g) dried chamomile flower	Combine all herbs; store in a glass jar.
½ ounce (14 g) dried wood betony	Make tea by the cup as needed: Steep
¼ ounce (7 g) dried St. John's wort	2 teaspoons (3 g) in 12 ounces (355 ml)
¼ ounce (7 g) dried angelica root	boiling water, covered, for 10 minutes.

STABLE MENOPAUSE MOOD CAPSULES

This formula isn't happy juice in a pill, but it's directed to balance the internal forces (such as fire and water) that are often in transition during Fulfillment.

Ingredients	Instructions
1 ounce (28 g) wild yam root powder	**YIELD:** 200 capsules
½ ounce (14 g) eleuthero root powder	Combine all ingredients in a bowl. Use the
¼ ounce (7 g) turmeric root powder	mixture to fill empty vegetable capsules.
¼ ounce (7 g) spirulina powder	Take 2 capsules twice daily.

COOL DOWN AND SLEEP TINCTURE

I typically recommend a tincture for nighttime waking, as the goal is to try to cling to any shred of sleep state versus waking up fully. A tincture is easy to keep next to the bed and take when half awake. Don't turn on a light; don't even open your eyes. Simply pick up the bottle, put 2 dropperfuls under your tongue, and lie back down.

Ingredients	Instructions
1 tablespoon (15 ml) hops tincture	**YIELD:** 1 ounce (28 ml)
1 teaspoon (5 ml) skullcap tincture	Combine all ingredients in a 1-ounce
¾ teaspoon (4 ml) chickweed tincture	(28 ml) amber dropper bottle.
½ teaspoon (3 ml) hawthorn leaf and flower tincture	Take 2 dropperfuls as needed.
½ teaspoon (3 ml) sage tincture	

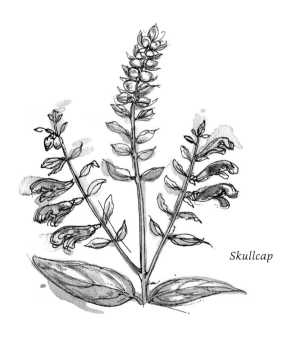

Skullcap

BRAIN SUPPORT

They say pregnancy brain is the worst, but I think anytime you have sudden dips and changes in hormones can challenge the thought processes. When it happens later in life, you can't help but wonder if it's the beginning of the end. Rest assured, it is not; it's just those lovely hormones forcing us to function differently. Here are some other questions to ask ourselves if the think tank isn't churning as well as it used to: Has my daily movement decreased? Is my circulation feeling strong? Am I eating enough? Am I getting enough sleep? Am I drinking enough water? These can all play a role in brain function and are worth giving attention to if needed.

Stock your home herbal pantry with the following for brain support:

Cayenne	Licorice root	Sage leaf
Dandelion root	Linden leaf and flower	Skullcap leaf
Ginkgo leaf	Lobelia leaf	Spirulina
Gotu Kola leaf	Nettle leaf	Turmeric root
Hawthorn leaf and flower	Rooibos	
	Rosemary leaf	

MEMORY TEA

This tea is a blend of herbs that all focus on mental acuity and clarity. Drink it as often as you'd like or before a work session to get your brain turned on.

½ ounce (14 g) dried gotu kola leaf	**YIELD:** 4 ounces (112 g)
½ ounce (14 g) dried skullcap leaf	Combine all herbs; store in a glass jar.
½ ounce (14 g) dried linden leaf and flower	Make tea by the cup as needed: Steep
½ ounce (14 g) dried rosemary leaf	2 teaspoons (3 g) in 12 ounces (355 ml)
½ ounce (14 g) dried sage leaf	of boiling water, covered, for 10 minutes.
1½ ounces (42 g) dried rooibos tea	

BRAIN BOOST CAPSULES

I'm a big believer in doing daily crossword puzzles to keep your brain sharp, but because I still have to Google the answers most of the time, I use these capsules daily to boost my brain's thinking power.

1 ounce (28 g) ginkgo leaf powder	YIELD: 200 capsules
½ ounce (14 g) rosemary leaf powder	Combine all ingredients in a bowl. Use
½ ounce (14 g) turmeric root powder	mixture to fill empty vegetable capsules.
¼ teaspoon ground cayenne pepper	Take 2 capsules twice daily.
	Note: Due to the cayenne, it is best to wear gloves to make these capsules.

BRAIN ALIVE TINCTURE

This is a great daily-use tincture to support your brain and circulation.

1½ teaspoons (8 ml) turmeric root tincture	YIELD: 1 ounce (28 ml)
1½ teaspoons (8 ml) spirulina tincture	Combine all ingredients in a 1-ounce
1½ teaspoons (8 ml) hawthorn leaf and flower tincture	(28 ml) amber dropper bottle. Take 1 dropperful 3 times per day.
½ teaspoon (3 ml) dandelion root tincture	
½ teaspoon (3 ml) nettle leaf tincture	
30 drops lobelia tincture	

THINK FAST! TINCTURE

We all have those days when our brain just isn't keeping up with us. Use this tincture as needed to jumpstart the brain back into action.

2 teaspoons (10 ml) rosemary tincture	YIELD: 1 ounce (28 ml)
1½ teaspoons (7 ml) licorice root tincture	Combine all ingredients in a 1-ounce
1¼ teaspoons (6 ml) ginkgo leaf tincture	(28 ml) amber dropper bottle. Take
1¼ teaspoons (6 ml) nettle leaf tincture	1 dropperful 3 times per day, as needed.
¼ teaspoon (1 ml) Cayenne tincture	

THINNING HAIR

Although losing hair is normal at different times of our lives, it's never comfortable for those experiencing it. Get a physical and consider asking your health care provider to check your thyroid to ensure you don't miss an overt cause of the problem. Boosting trace minerals, scalp massage, and reducing stress are all key to treatment.

Stock your home herbal pantry with the following for thinning hair:

Ginkgo leaf	Kelp	Rosemary leaf
Green tea	Nettle leaf	Schizandra berry
Horsetail	Reishi mushroom	Spirulina

VITAL GREENS CAPSULES

Packed with vitamins and minerals, this blend supports the body on almost every level. When you offer the body an abundance of nutrition, the hair benefits.

½ ounce (14 g) spirulina powder

½ ounce (14 g) schizandra berry powder

¼ ounce (7 g) horsetail powder

¼ ounce (7 g) nettle leaf powder

¼ ounce (7 g) kelp powder

¼ ounce (7 g) reishi mushroom powder

YIELD: 200 capsules

Combine all ingredients in a bowl. Use the mixture to fill empty vegetable capsules. Take 2 capsules twice daily for 6 to 8 weeks.

SCALP MASSAGE OIL

They say rubbing the scalp stimulates the hair follicles to grow. Put some oil onto your scalp and look at yourself in the mirror. Massage the oil down to the scalp and move the scalp back and forth and side to side for 5 minutes a day.

½ ounce (14 g) dried Rosemary leaf

½ ounce (14 g) dried nettle leaf

½ ounce (14 g) dried green tea

½ ounce (14 g) dried ginkgo

Olive oil

YIELD: 1 to 1½ cups (235 to 355 ml)

Preheat oven to 170°F (77°C). Place herbs in a glass baking dish and pour enough olive oil over them to cover by 1 to 2 inches (3 to 5 cm). Bake for 4 hours. Allow oil to cool and then strain into a squeeze bottle for easy application. Squirt close to the scalp over the entire head. Massage for 15 minutes; better yet, get someone else to massage it for you. Apply 3 to 4 times per week.

PROLAPSE

Whether it's in the bladder or uterus, the feeling of prolapse is one of a deep dragging weight in the lower abdomen. As we age, or after pregnancy, our ligaments tend to stretch and no longer support our structures as they once did. Ligaments are difficult to nourish, as they do not have a direct blood supply to feed them. They are dependent on fluids washing over them to give them what they need to uphold their integrity. Uterus and bladder ligaments are also dependent on estrogen to stay strong. Uterine prolapse is when the uterus drops into the vaginal canal; bladder prolapse is when the bladder drops into the vaginal canal.

PROLAPSE TINCTURE

This formula can be used for either the uterus or the bladder to support and tone the ligaments.

1 tablespoon (15 ml) uva ursi leaf tincture

1 tablespoon (15 ml) red raspberry leaf tincture

2 teaspoons (10 ml) horse chestnut tincture

2 teaspoons (10 ml) dandelion root tincture

2 teaspoons (10 ml) horsetail leaf tincture

YIELD: 2 ounces (60 ml)

Combine all ingredients in a 2-ounce (60 ml) amber dropper bottle.
Take 1 dropperful 3 times per day for 8 weeks.

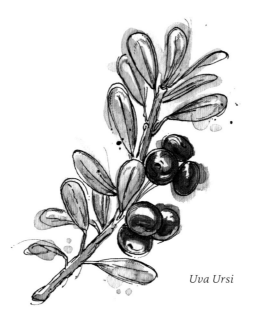

Uva Ursi

CASTOR OIL TREATMENT FOR PROLAPSE

Treatment from the outside in is a good idea when trying to support core supportive structures of the body.

Ingredients	Instructions
2 tablespoons (18 g) cracked horse chestnuts 2 tablespoons (28 g) comfrey leaf 1 tablespoon (9 g) red raspberry leaf 1 to 1½ cups (235 to 355 ml) castor oil	YIELD: 1 cup (235 ml) Preheat oven to 170°F (77°C). Place herbs in a glass baking dish and pour enough castor oil over them to cover by 1 to 2 inches (3 to 5 cm). Bake for 6 hours. Allow to cool and then strain the mixture into a storage container. Rub 2 to 3 teaspoons (10 to 15 ml) over the lower abdomen daily for 8 to 12 weeks.

Dr. Christopher recommends using a douche of equal parts chaparral, elderflowers, and peppermint leaf. I would also recommend seeking out a Mayan abdominal practitioner for an abdominal treatment. Pelvic floor work would also be advised. Just like at any time of your life, caring for your body takes energy and dedication.

When we get older, it becomes more apparent when we don't take care of ourselves. Our physical ability to compensate for the errors of our ways—rich foods, lack of exercise and water, and increased stress—has been diminished. But this also can be one of the best times of any women's life, should you choose it. Self-care through balanced nutrition, herbal medicine, body movement, and positive thinking will have powerful effects and create the best you. Feeling good on the inside makes you glow on the outside.

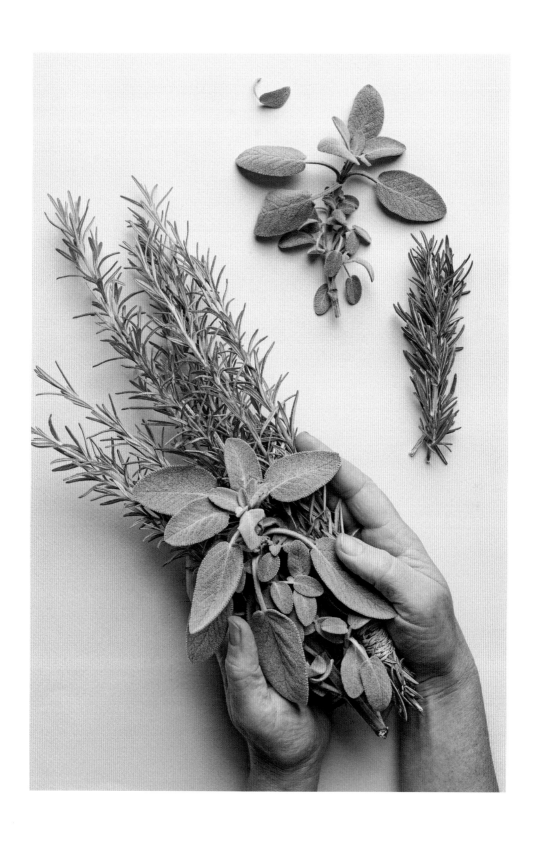

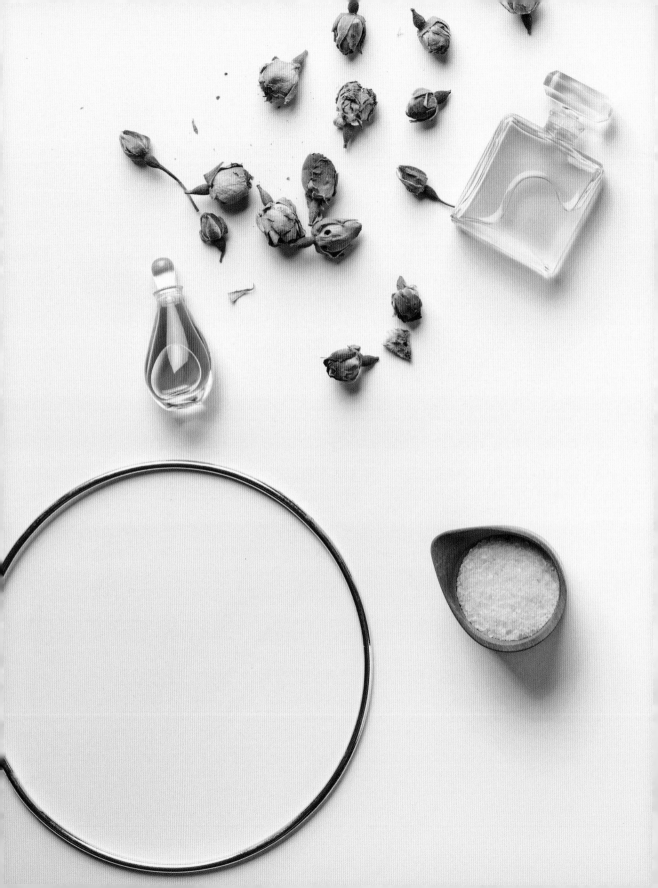

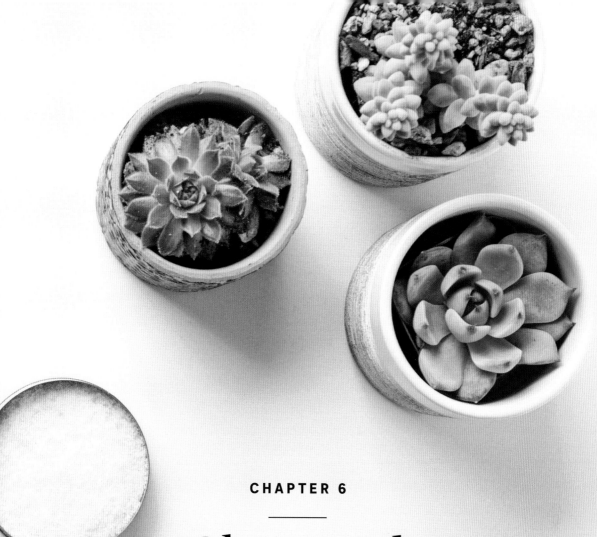

CHAPTER 6

Skin and Body Health

CELEBRATE THE SKIN YOU'RE IN. There is nothing wrong with wanting to look and feel your best. The key is to love yourself from the inside out. Our body is a temporary temple. If you give it attention and plenty of self-care, it will excel in form, function, and beauty. There is nothing more important than feeling good on the inside. This is the first step to being radiant on the surface. But it goes deeper than that. Your emotional terrain plays a big part in not only how your body functions on the inside but also what you are showing on the outside. I sometimes use the phrase "Fake it until you make it." This doesn't mean put on a happy face and ignore the troubles you are encountering. It means that life is filled with difficult situations; be aware of them, have some sort of strategy in place to improve or grow from them, and be sure to balance difficulties with day-to-day joy. If you stay in the misery or doom and gloom, you could be imprinting that onto your physical health and outward appearance.

Remember that the skin is the largest organ of the body. It works day and night to keep you protected, releasing what is necessary, regulating your body temperature, and managing the multitude of sensations you are perpetually interpreting from the external world. My mom tried her best to teach me to care for my skin as a child, but I didn't have time for such practices. I didn't care about going to bed with dirt from the backyard on my face or wearing sunscreen. I was young and my skin would last forever. Ha! Your skin is a precious protective organ, one that should be nourished and cared for like any other body part.

The skin's internal partner is the liver. As we've discussed, the liver is master detoxifier, taking the day's worth of by-products and breaking them down to be recycled, reabsorbed, or released. When the liver gets bogged down, the skin always offers to take up the slack. This may result in acne or skin eruptions as the skin takes some of the detoxifying load off the liver and pushes it out through the skin. The same can go for the lymphatic system. If congestion gets to be too much, the skin may begin to pull from the glands to relieve the overload.

Nighttime is when the liver clocks in for work. It uses our sleep time to cleanse the body in preparation for the next day. This is the time when everything else is shut down, giving the liver full reign of the energy it needs to do its best. So here is something to think about: When you eat late at night, energy is needed then for the digestion process. Your energy is diverted from the liver to digestion. Not only that, the liver has to wait until the digestion process is complete to fully begin its work.

This results in a shortened overnight detox time, meaning the liver begins to fall behind. If this pattern is repeated, it's easy to see how the liver begins to get overwhelmed and rely on other bodily functions to help support the body's detoxification pathways.

Another consideration is not sleeping long enough. Research has proven the myriad reasons sleep is vital to our health. It is during sleep that the liver does its work. If you shorten your sleep cycle to five hours, you are most likely shortening the detoxification cycle, which can cause buildup or congestion down the road. That said, if you stay up late once in a while, don't worry; this is more about long-term patterns.

We must also think about hormone health and digestion (see chapter 3, chapter 5, and chapter 7) when thinking of the radiance of the skin. Chronic inflammation, poor gut flora, food allergies, and stress can all lead to digestive disruption, which can result in uneven or blemished skin. The same goes for hormonal imbalance. Learning about and understanding your hormonal patterns (and perhaps imbalance) will help you to know which herbs are best to correct the underlying disharmony that may be affecting your skin.

First, initiate a daily ritual for yourself and your body. Find a place you can sit quietly for a few minutes each day. Maybe it's before you get out of bed or before you fall asleep. Maybe there is a place in your house or backyard that provides you peace and relaxation. Wherever and whenever it is, get comfortable and take three deep inhalations. Then start at the top of your head and run your hands slowly and gently all over your body. With each new body part, take a deep breath and give thanks for all your body does for you. Each day, you wake up and do extraordinary things. You may not think so, but it's true. Give your body the thanks it deserves. It'll respond in kind.

Using the following recipes is another way to say thank you. Incorporate them into your daily or life routine, or use them in ritual for deeper connection to yourself and your body. By taking the time to connect to your body through self-care, you unlock the magnificence that resides within.

Our faces have been the crux of purity, vanity, and cruelty since the dawn of time. No other body part is judged, dissected, manipulated, or valued as much as the human face, particularly the female face. It is as simple as this: You were born beautiful. Don't let anyone take that away from you or tempt you to think otherwise.

I can honestly say I've never met a smile that hasn't made me smile in return. Wouldn't it be amazing if we were looked at through our smiles? Alas, we are not, and that puts a lot of pressure on people of all types to be beautiful. I dare you to focus on creating beauty from the inside out. We are fortunate to live in a time in which beauty is finally being allowed to take many different forms. The more we allow this process, the happier our world will be.

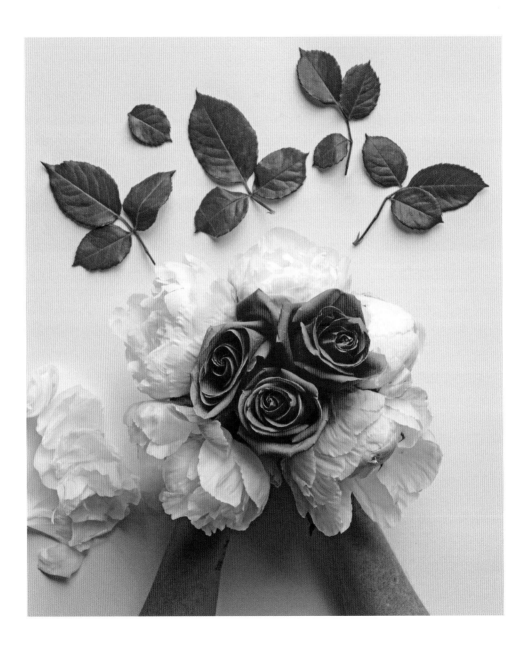

FACIAL SKIN

The skin on your face is the most exposed skin on your body, with your hands coming in at a close second. We often don't realize the onslaught of various exposures our face faces every day. Sun is just one of the hazards; there are also air pollution, wind, rain, snow, heat and cooling machine particles, dust, pollen, and I'm sure much more. As I write this, we are experiencing some of the worst wildfires in Oregon's history. Each morning and night, I wash my face and can't believe the amount of ash that is present despite the fires being a great distance away. Even if your face doesn't appear dirty, after a day of living, you can bet it is.

HERBAL FOAM FACE CLEANSER

Use each morning and night to clear impediments away and start fresh. It's best for normal to sensitive skin.

½ cup (120 ml) chickweed, plantain, and chamomile herbal infusion (Add 1 teaspoon [1.5 g] of each herb to 8 ounces [235 ml] water; steep overnight and strain.)

2 tablespoons (30 ml) jojoba oil

2 tablespoons (30 ml) rosehip oil

2 teaspoons (10 ml) aloe vera gel

20 drops frankincense essential oil or lemon essential oil, or 10 drops each

½ cup (120 ml) unscented liquid castile soap

YIELD: 1 cup (235 ml)

Mix together all ingredients except the castile soap. Check the scent and adjust if necessary to your liking.

Slowly stir in castile soap. If using a blender or mixer, turn it on a very low setting; otherwise it'll be a foaming explosion. Transfer mixture to a pump soap bottle and give it a try. If is it too thick, add just a touch of water. No need to remix and shake.

Variation: OIL-RICH SKIN FACIAL FOAM CLEANSER

Replace rosehip oil with grapeseed oil. Use myrrh, tea tree, and ylang-ylang essential oils, 8 drops each to start, instead of frankincense and lemon. Prepare as above.

Variation: DRY SKIN FACIAL FOAM CLEANSER

Replace rosehip oil with avocado oil. Use geranium, cedarwood, and rose essential oils, 8 drops each to start, instead of frankincense and lemon. Prepare as above.

LET'S GO DEEP FACIAL CLEANSER

If you are looking to go a little deeper in your cleaning routine, try this formula, which utilizes charcoal to pull out lower level buildup.

½ cup (109 g) organic coconut oil

½ cup (120 ml) plantain herbal oil

¼ ounce (7 g) charcoal powder

2 tablespoons (28 g) organic activated baking soda

10 drops grapefruit essential oil

5 drops cedarwood essential oil

3 drops juniper essential oil

YIELD: 1 cup (235 ml)

Gently heat the coconut oil over low heat if it isn't already in a liquid state. Once it is, turn off the heat and combine with the plantain herbal oil, charcoal powder, and baking soda. Add the essential oils and adjust the scent by 2 or 3 drops if desired. Transfer to a storage container. When ready to use, warm and moisten your face with a washcloth. Massage a small amount of cleanser over your entire face, avoiding the eyes, nostrils, and mouth. This does a great job of removing makeup; just use it gently, and remove it quickly if you use it on your eyes. You can let it rest on your face for a few minutes and then remove using warm water and a washcloth.

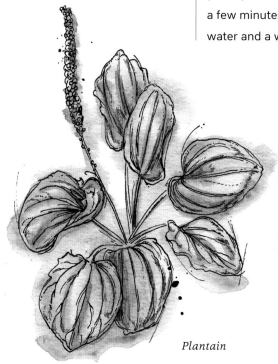

Plantain

HERBAL OIL CLEANSER

Oil dissolves oil. Many people find that using an oil cleanser not only reduces breakouts but also softens the skin and promotes a healthy glow. The best way to fully utilize an oil cleanser is to first apply it to dry skin and then steam your face. This can be easily accomplished in the shower; just leave it on while you wash your hair or body, then rinse it off. Or apply a moderately hot washcloth to your face for a minute before rinsing. I've also found that rinsing my face with warm water before applying the cleanser works.

NORMAL SKIN: ARGAN FLOWER POWER OIL CLEANSER

1 teaspoon (1.5 g) dried chamomile flowers	**YIELD:** 4 ounces (120 ml)
1 teaspoon (1.5 g) dried red clover blossoms	Preheat oven to 170°F (77°C). Place
1 teaspoon (1.5 g) dried rose petals	herbs in a small glass dish, cover with
½ cup (120 ml) argan oil	oil, and bake for 4 hours. Strain and
10 drops geranium, carrot seed, cypress, or lemongrass essential oil (optional, for longevity of product)	transfer to an amber bottle with a dropper. Add essential oil, if using.

OIL-RICH SKIN: GREEN GODDESS OIL CLEANSER

1 teaspoon (1.5 g) dried plantain leaf	**YIELD:** 4 ounces (120 ml)
1 teaspoon (1.5 g) dried thyme leaf	Preheat oven to 170°F (77°C). Place herbs
1 teaspoon (1.5 g) dried calendula flower	in a small glass dish, cover with oil, and
½ cup (120 ml) grapeseed oil	bake for 4 hours. Strain and transfer to
10 drops chamomile, ylang-ylang, or clary sage essential oil (optional, for longevity of product)	an amber bottle with a dropper. Add essential oil, if using.

DRY SKIN: LET IT RAIN OIL CLEANSER

1 teaspoon (1.5 g) dried comfrey leaf	**YIELD:** 4 ounces (120 ml)
1 teaspoon (1.5 g) dried rose petals	Preheat oven to 170°F (77°C). Place herbs
1 teaspoon (1.5 g) dried marshmallow root	in a small glass dish, cover with oil, and
½ cup (120 ml) hemp oil	bake for 4 hours. Strain and transfer to
10 drops patchouli, neroli, or rose essential oil (optional, for longevity of product)	an amber bottle with a dropper. Add essential oil, if using.

MIRACLE GRAINS

One of my favorite herb teachers, Rosemary Gladstar, first introduced me to using grains to wash my face almost twenty-five years ago. At the time, I was a newly enthusiastic herbal initiate, and despite how my mother had tried unsuccessfully to get me to care for my face, I basically tried everything Rosemary recommended. Washing grains are nothing new; having been used throughout the world in various cultures, they are most often concocted from elements that are readily available. A word of caution here: "Microbeads," which are a common ingredient in commercial scrubs and body products, are toxic and are wreaking havoc on the environment. They are not biodegradable and are often released into our oceans, becoming a direct source of pollution and hazard to all ocean wildlife. Please reconsider purchasing these products and try any of the following recipes as a wonderful substitute.

1 cup (115 g) powdered French green clay, bentonite clay (has more drawing power), or red clay

½ cup (38 g) finely ground dry brown rice or dry beans (Adzuki is a common choice.)

¼ cup (50 g) fine sea salt or sugar

¼ cup baking soda (45 g) or ground chia seeds (41 g)

3 tablespoons (14 g) finely ground rose petals, lavender flowers, and/or orange peel

YIELD: 2 cups (262 g)

Ensuring each ingredient is finely ground, mix all ingredients together and store in a dry glass jar.

To use: Pour a small amount into your palm and mix in a few drops of warm water until a paste forms. Gently rub in a circular motion all around your face. Rinse with warm water.

HERBAL FACIAL SERUM

Facial serums have become very poplar, and I can't deny that I love them as much as my face does. A serum, by definition, is a lightweight moisturizer that penetrates deeper to deliver active ingredients into your skin. Unlike creams and lotions, which are richer and create a barrier on top of the skin, serums dive to the skin's deeper depths.

1 drop helichrysum essential oil

1 drop sandalwood essential oil

2 drops frankincense essential oil

1 ounce (28 ml) rose petal-infused jojoba oil

YIELD: 1 ounce (28 ml)

Combine essential oils in a 1-ounce (28 ml) glass amber bottle with dropper. Add infused jojoba oil. Close bottle and gently invert a few times to blend. I use 5 to 10 drops after I wash my face, twice daily.

VARIATIONS: DIFFERENT CARRIER OILS

Using different carrier oils to infuse the rose petals lets you personalize your serum. Here is a quick guide to carrier oils.

Normal skin: Coconut, hemp, grapeseed, sweet almond

Dry skin: Sweet almond, rosehip, avocado, olive, evening primrose

Sensitive skin: Jojoba, sweet almond, apricot, sesame seed, kukui nut, avocado

Oil-rich skin: Jojoba, grapeseed, sweet almond, apricot, neem

Mature skin: Rosehip, jojoba, sweet almond, apricot, hemp, kukui nut, sea buckthorn, tamanu

Combination skin: Argan, grapeseed, jojoba, evening primrose, sweet almond, apricot, macadamia nut

Facial Masks

HERBAL FACIAL MASKS

Facial masks are a great way to get an instant facial glow. I often wonder why I don't do them more often, as I look so good afterward! My dear friend Tatianna is the queen of facial masks. When we were roommates, it was never a surprise to see her whipping up various herbal and food concoctions to put onto her face. Most were wildly successful, with only a couple epic fails. It can't be denied; masks offer incredible moisture to the face, as well as detoxification, increased circulation, and the reupping of vital face nutrients.

1 cup (115 g) French green clay

1 teaspoon (1.5 g) dried lavender

1 teaspoon (1.5 g) dried rose

1 teaspoon (1.5 g) dried chamomile flowers

YIELD: 1 cup (115 g)

Combine all ingredients; put in a glass storage container.

To use: Place 2 to 4 teaspoons (3 to 6 g) of the mixture in a bowl and add enough hot water to make a paste. Apply gently to the face and neck. Leave on for 10 to 15 minutes. Wash away with warm water and a washcloth.

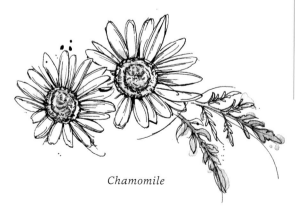

Chamomile

FINDING BALANCE FACIAL MASK

Whether your face tends to be dry, oily, or somewhere in between, this face mask has a sweet spot for you.

1 teaspoon (5 ml) aloe vera juice

1 teaspoon (2.2 g) turmeric powder

1 teaspoon (7 g) honey

YIELD: 1 face mask

Mix all ingredients until smooth. Apply to the face and leave on for 10 to 15 minutes. Wash away with warm water and a washcloth.

MINERAL FACE-LIFT

Using herbal minerals to improve your skin's glow and texture is like getting a mini face-lift right at home.

½ teaspoon (1.5 g) ground mullein leaf or power

½ teaspoon (1.5 g) ground red raspberry leaf or powder

½ teaspoon (1.5 g) alfalfa leaf or powder

¼ cup (60 ml) castor oil

½ teaspoon (2.5 ml) lemon juice

YIELD: 1 face mask

Mix all 3 powders together. Add castor oil and lemon juice; blend well. Apply to the face and leave on for 10 to 15 minutes. Wash away with warm water and a washcloth.

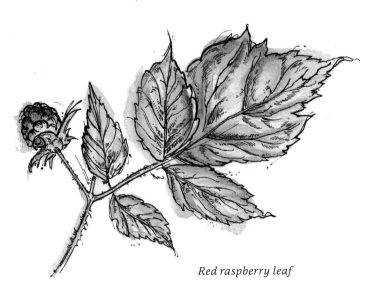

Red raspberry leaf

Facial Steaming

Facial steaming is a great way to open up the skin and purify the pores. Using gentle heat with steam, you can add moisture to your face. Please be very careful with steaming if you haven't done it before. Ensure that the heat and steam are a comfortable temperature. Steaming should be pleasant; there should never be a feeling that your face is burning off. Also, be sure to let the steam breathe off for a moment on a pot before you stick your face in there. We're rewarding your skin, not cooking it.

ROSE OASIS FACIAL STEAM

Want to have a rosy glow? The gentle steam of rose petals nourishes the skin to baby-like softness. It's a great activity to do with your friends.

1 ounce (28 g) dried rose petals

20 drops rose essential oil

YIELD: 1 facial steam treatment

Bring 4 quarts (4 L) water to an almost boil; add rose petals. Turn off the heat and cover tightly; let sit for 15 minutes. Open the lid and quickly add rose essential oil. Close the lid again for 2 minutes.

Carry the pot to a safe place—not on the stove—where you can easily lean over into the steam. Open the lid and let steam breathe off. Be sure long hair is tied back and that all hair is off your face. (Use a headband or cloth to lift your hair away from your face.) Take turns leaning into the steam for short stints to get a nice heat to the face and a bit of sweat. Take care not to overheat or burn your face. You can use a towel over your head to "hold in" the steam. Steam for 15 to 20 minutes and then rinse your face with warm water.

GREEN TEA FACIAL STEAM

This wonderful steam is high in antioxidants to help your face glow and feel ultra-smooth.

¼ ounce (7 g) green tea, or 4 tea bags (Any green tea will do.)

2 tablespoons (18 g) dried lemongrass

YIELD: 1 facial steam treatment

Bring 5 cups (1.2 L) of water to an almost boil; add green tea and lemongrass. Turn off the heat and cover tightly. Let steep for 5 minutes. Steam for 10 to 15 minutes; relax and enjoy.

THE FRESHEN UP FACIAL STEAM

Bringing you bright and shiny feelings and facial glow!

1 teaspoon (1 g) fresh or dried basil

1 teaspoon (1 g) fresh or dried mint

1 teaspoon (1 g) fresh or dried rosemary

1 teaspoon (1 g) fresh or dried lavender

YIELD: 1 facial steam treatment

Bring 5 cups (1.2 L) of water to an almost boil; add all herbs. Turn off the heat and cover tightly. Let steep for 5 minutes. Steam for 10 to 15 minutes; relax and enjoy.

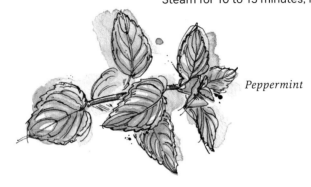

Peppermint

Toners

Facial toners have two purposes. First, they balance pH and remove those last traces of impurity from the skin. Second, they give me a sensation I'm addicted to. I love the bright, cool tingle on my skin. I often imagine I'm on the deck of a boat getting spritzed by the ocean waves. Yes, I grew up in the Sea Breeze facial toner era! Luckily, we can now all make our own from beautiful ingredients that truly support our skin.

BEAUTY AT ANY AGE FACIAL TONER

This toner is great for all skin types and ages.

4 ounces (120 ml) rose hydrosol

2 ounces (60 ml) herb infusion (Place 1 tea-spoon [1.5 g] comfrey leaf, 1 teaspoon [1.5 g] borage leaf, 1 teaspoon [1.5 g] rosemary leaf, and
¼ teaspoon turmeric root or powder in 5 ounces [150 ml] hot water; let steep for 1 hour, then strain.)

2 ounces (60 ml) witch hazel extract

30 drops grapefruit essential oil

15 drops peppermint essential oil

YIELD: 8 ounces (235 ml)

Combine rose hydrosol, herb infusion, and witch hazel extract; transfer to an 8-ounce (235 ml) spray bottle. Add grape-fruit and peppermint essential oils. Shake well before each use. Spray onto face; use a cotton pad to remove.

PURITY FACIAL TONER

This toner is geared to leave the face clear of excess oils and promote evenness of skin.

2 teaspoons (3 g) dried lemon peel	YIELD: 4 ounces (120 ml)
2 teaspoons (3 g) dried rosemary leaf	Place herbs into witch hazel extract and let steep
2 teaspoons (3 g) dried plantain leaf	for 2 weeks. Keep in a cool dark place during
4 ounces (120 ml) witch hazel extract	steeping, shaking every day. Strain and transfer to a
10 drops myrrh essential oil	clean 4-ounce (120 ml) spray bottle. Add myrrh and
7 drops melissa essential oil	melissa essential oils. Shake well before each use.
	Spray onto the face; use a cotton pad to remove.

VARIATION: GET CREATIVE WITH YOUR TONER!

One of the great gifts of herbs is that you can customize everything to your specific needs. Look below and learn which different ingredients you can use to blend your perfect toner. By no means are these lists exclusive.

Toner foundation: Witch hazel, apple cider vinegar, distilled water, hydrosols

Great herbs for skin toners: Rose, sage, yarrow, comfrey, thyme, rosemary, calendula, plantain, borage, peppermint, lavender, chamomile, echinacea, red raspberry

Essential oils: Grapefruit, melissa, peppermint, sage, lavender, lemon, myrrh, cedar, chamomile, helichrysum, frankincense, sandalwood

Facial Glow Spa Treatment

One of my favorite things to do is gather friends, both women and men, and have a relaxing group spa day. They are often in winter, when I can turn on the fire and hot drinks abound, but summer sessions have been known to happen as well. Whether you are with friends or it's a quiet spa experience for one, this regimen is one of my favorites.

Start by having a warm face-washing session. Using your favorite cleanser, spend a good three to four minutes washing your face. Pat it dry and then use washing grains to really release all the old and allow the new to shine. Next, give the oil cleanser a try. Be sure to use two to three hot towels on your face to really heat up the oil. After rinsing this off, a fresh mask of roses, chamomile, and mint feels heavenly. Sip some tea while thinking about nothing for fifteen minutes. After rinsing, apply facial serum slowly and deliberately while saying the mantra "You are so beautiful" (because you are!). End with a little spritz to the face of rose and geranium water.

HANDS

I've been intrigued by hands my whole life. I have a series of photographs of my family members' hands because to me they tell the full stories of their lives. All the spots, wrinkles, scars, and interesting attributes seem to say as much when I look at these photos. When I look at my sister's hands, I am always in awe. Even though she's older than I am, her hands still retain the milky smooth tone of an Italian countess who's never done a day's worth of work. Mind you, my sister has worked plenty, but she has always—and I mean always—taken care of her hands. My hands, on the other hand, have been a bit neglected. They are often stained with dirt, mud, or some random plant material. If I ever do end up doing something special for them, it's rubbing them with the dredges of this or that herbal product that I happen to be making. Whether you are like me or my sister, below are some great recipes to show your hands the extra love they deserve.

LADY OF THE GARDEN SALVE

This is a hardworking, deep-penetrating salve to soften up even the hardest of farmer's hands.

⅛ ounce (3.5 g) plantain leaf

⅛ ounce (3.5 g) comfrey leaf

⅛ ounce (3.5 g) calendula flower

⅛ ounce (3.5 g) horsetail leaf

1 cup (235 ml) olive oil

1 teaspoon (5 ml) vitamin E oil

1 ounce (28 g) beeswax

10 drops frankincense essential oil

10 drops chamomile essential oil

YIELD: 8 ounces (235 ml)

Preheat oven to 170°F (77°C). Place herbs in a glass baking dish and cover with olive oil. Bake for 4 hours. Strain. Add vitamin E oil. Transfer oil to a saucepan and heat over low heat; add beeswax, stirring until completely melted. Add frankincense and chamomile essential oils. Pour into a storage container of choice and use daily. I keep mine in my garden.

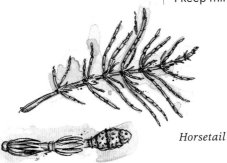

Horsetail

BRIGHT HANDS CREAM

This is a cream to brighten dark spots and even out the texture of your hands.

½ ounce (14 g) dried chamomile flowers

½ ounce (14 g) dried lady's mantle leaf

½ ounce (14 g) dried lemon balm leaf

¾ cup (175 ml) sweet almond oil

2 tablespoons (28 g) beeswax

1 cup (218 g) shea butter

20 drops cedarwood essential oil

20 drops lemongrass essential oil

YIELD: 8 ounces (235 ml)

Preheat oven to 170°F (77°C). Place herbs in a glass baking dish place and cover with almond oil. Bake for 4 hours. Strain. Measure ¾ cup (175 ml) of sweet almond oil into a saucepan. Add beeswax and shea butter; heat on low setting, stirring to melt the beeswax. Let cool for 3 to 5 minutes. Add cedarwood and lemongrass essential oils. Transfer to a storage container.

SMOOTH AS SILK HAND CREAM

This recipe uses a combination of butters, oils, and waters. The key is in the emulsification step, which allows all three to blend together into a luscious cream. This recipe may seem to have a lot of steps, but I assure you it's much easier than you think, and the outcome is worth the work.

BUTTERS:

½ ounce (14 g) beeswax by weight

¾ ounce (21 g) coconut oil by weight

½ ounce (14 g) shea butter by weight

OILS:

¼ cup (60 ml) avocado oil

¼ cup (60 ml) rosehip seed oil

¼ cup (60 ml) calendula-infused grapeseed oil

1 tablespoon (15 ml) carrot seed oil

1 tablespoon (15 ml) vitamin E oil

WATERS:

⅓ cup (80 ml) rose or lavender hydrosol

⅓ cup (80 ml) aloe vera gel

40 drops essential oil of your choosing: rose, lavender, lemongrass, or frankincense

YIELD: 12 ounces (352 g)

Gently warm beeswax, coconut oil, and shea butter in a double boiler or a Pyrex measuring cup submerged in a pan of hot water. Use the lowest heat possible, even though it takes longer. Stir continuously as the mixture melts and blends the oils together.

In a separate bowl, combine avocado, rosehip seed, calendula, carrot seed, and vitamin E oils. Once the first oils are melted, turn the heat off and slowly add the other oils to combine. You may notice that the beeswax begins to harden as it cools. If it gets too thick, turn the heat back on just enough to melt everything again. You don't

(continued)

want the oils to be too hot for many reasons, one being that the mixture has to cool a bit before you add the water for it to emulsify properly.

After all the oils are mixed, transfer the mixture to a blender or bowl; allow it to cool until it is no longer translucent and takes on a waxy appearance. At this point, you are ready to add the waters (the hydrosol and aloe vera gel). Begin blending on high speed, or whipping quickly if doing it by hand; slowly add the waters. If you are doing this by hand, you'll need to have a helper add the waters so that you can whip continuously. It should emulsify in 2 to 3 minutes, creating a cream. Add the essential oils last; mix briefly. Transfer to a sterile storage jar and label.

Because of the vitamin E and essential oils, this cream should last for 6 to 8 months.

My favorite part? Taking the remnants from the blender and rubbing them all up and down my arms and legs.

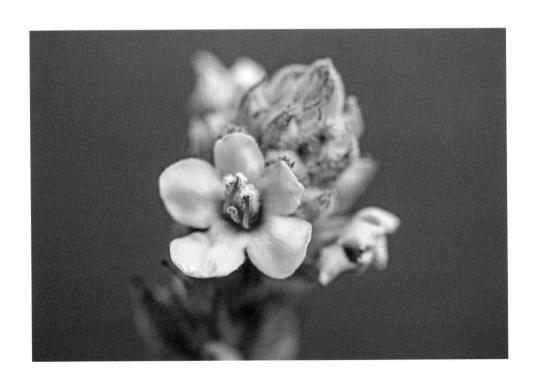

NAIL HEALTH

I've gone through many cycles with my nail care practices. Sometimes, I get manicures regularly, more for the cuticle maintenance than anything else; at other times, I have a regular routine of home care. I love the look and feel of nonpainted, well-cared-for fingernails. They look so healthy and clean!

DIY NAIL STRENGTHENING POLISH

This natural nail strengthener has high mineral content that catapults the growth of fingernails. It's a good formula for treating nail fungus as well.

¼ ounce (7 g) dried horsetail herb	YIELD: 4 ounces (120 ml)
¼ ounce (7 g) dried nettle leaf	Preheat oven to 170°F (77°C). Place herbs in a glass baking dish and pour castor oil over them. Bake for 6 hours. Strain. Transfer to a 4-ounce (120 ml) amber bottle with dropper. Add essential oils and shake well. Apply once daily to each nail to promote nail growth, health, and strength.
¾ cup (175 ml) castor oil	
10 drops lemon essential oil	
10 drops lavender essential oil	
10 drops myrrh essential oil	

CUTICLE RESCUE OIL

The health of your cuticles affects the health of your nails. Use this oil to soften and then remove the older cuticle.

¼ ounce (7 g) dried rose petals	YIELD: 8 ounces (235 ml)
¼ ounce (7 g) dried calendula	Preheat oven to 170°F (77°C). Place herbs in a glass baking dish and pour almond oil over them. Bake for 6 hours. Strain. Add vitamin E oil. Add essential oils. Heat 2 ounces (60 ml) of your creation and pour into a bowl. Find a quiet, comfortable place to sit and submerge your fingertips in the warm oil. Relax for as long as you can; then, massage your fingertips before removing your hands. Use cuticle trimmers to trim away older cuticle. Wipe your hands clean with a towel and marvel at the effects of such a simple treatment. If your hands were clean before your treatment, you can reuse the oil.
¼ ounce (7 g) dried chamomile	
1 cup (235 ml) sweet almond oil	
1 teaspoon (5 ml) vitamin E oil	
10 drops lavender essential oil	
10 drops lemon essential oil.	

HAIR HEALTH

Our hair is an energetic thing. It takes in emotions, experiences, and outside exposures. There is also a genetic component to how our hair looks that we can't escape. Our health plays an equal role in the state of our hair. It's no wonder we cut, color, grow, and cut it again. Focusing on the health perspective, if you are nourished and hydrated, it's most likely your hair is showing it. If you are on the other end of the spectrum—overworked, stressed, and eating sporadically—well, that takes a toll on your hair. Luckily, there are numerous herbs high in minerals and vitamins to give your hair the boost it may need.

GROW ON HAIR TONIC

For those wishing for a little extra length, use this tonic 2 to 3 times per week.

2 tablespoons (9 g) dried rosemary

2 tablespoons (9 g) dried nettle

2 tablespoons (9 g) dried alfalfa leaf

YIELD: 1 quart (946 ml)

Bring 1 quart (946 ml) of water almost to a boil. Add herbs. Cover and let steep overnight. Strain.

After shampooing, rinse your hair with this tonic, massaging it into the scalp. Ideally, leave it on for 15 minutes before rinsing out.

SHINY LOCKS TONIC

Use these herbs to improve your hair's gloss and natural shine.

2 tablespoons (9 g) dried parsley

2 tablespoons (9 g) dried rosemary

2 tablespoons (9 g) dried nettle leaf

1 quart (946 ml) apple cider vinegar

YIELD: 1 quart (946 ml)

Add all herbs to the apple cider vinegar. Seal and let steep for 2 weeks. Strain.

After shampooing, rinse your hair with 4 ounces (120 ml) of tonic, massaging it into the scalp. It can be used every time you wash your hair.

GRAY GRAY GO AWAY HAIR TONIC

How did the fo-ti herb (*Polygonum multiflorum*) get its Chinese name, *He Shou Wu*? There once was a general named He who was convicted of a crime. He was sentenced to a dug-out cell deep in the ground and given no food or water, basically to await his death. One year later, guards returned to collect his remains, and low and behold, he was still alive! Not only that, his hair had turned back to black. He was strong and had been surviving off the root of the one vine that grew deep in the crevices of the cell, the fo-ti root. Folklore perhaps, but I have personally seen fo-ti transform gray hair to black when taken internally in the form of tea or capsule. Drinking 2 to 3 cups of fo-ti tea per day, or taking 4 fo-ti capsules 3 times per day, supports the liver, kidneys, and reproductive organs and increases vitality and stamina. This tonic, meanwhile, utilizes fo-ti's ability to get rid of gray hair!

½ ounce (14 g) rosemary leaf

½ ounce (14 g) fo-ti

½ ounce (14 g) tea, depending on hair color: black tea for darker shades, chamomile for blonds, and rooibos for red tones

YIELD: 2 cups (475 ml)

Steep herbs in 2 cups (475 ml) hot water overnight. Strain. To use, mix the infusion with 1 to 2 tablespoons (14 to 28 g) coconut oil and apply to wet hair. Let it sit on your hair for at least 1 hour, wrapped in a towel. Rinse with cool water.

Other Herbs for Gray Hair Treatment

- **Dark Hair:** Rosemary, sage, nettle, cloves, cinnamon, black walnut hulls, comfrey root
- **Blond Hair:** Chamomile, calendula, lemon peel, saffron, marigold, yarrow, sunflower petals, mullein flowers
- **Red Hair:** Hibiscus flowers, red clover, rosehips, red rose petals, beets, carrots, marigold

FLAKY SCALP TREATMENT

Don't be discouraged by dry scalp. Although taking essential fatty acids and drinking more water are said to help, the water, shampoos, and treatments we put onto our scalp often lead to dryness. This treatment helps combat them.

Ingredients	Instructions
1 ounce (28 g) dried lemon peel 1 ounce (28 g) dried burdock root ½ ounce (14 g) fresh thyme ½ ounce (14 g) fresh parsley 16 ounces (475 ml) apple cider vinegar	YIELD: 16 ounces (475 ml) Let herbs soak in the apple cider vinegar for 2 weeks, shaking daily. Strain and store in a spray bottle. Two or 3 times per week, spray down hair after shampooing and let sit for 15 minutes. You should notice a decrease in flakes after 1 to 2 weeks.

In-Grown Hair Solutions

SPOT TREATMENT

For spot treatment of in-grown hairs, try this; follow up with the scrub below.

Ingredients	Instructions
½ ounce (14 g) plantain leaf powder ¼ ounce (7 g) bentonite clay powder Evening primrose oil	YIELD: 1 ounce (28 g) Mix powders with just enough evening primrose oil to make a paste. Apply as a spot treatment to draw out ingrown hairs. Leave on for 10 to 15 minutes.

SUGAR SCRUB

Inflammation from shaving or waxing can be a real annoyance, especially along the bikini line. Use this gentle scrub to help reduce discomfort and discourage future in-grown hairs.

Ingredients	Instructions
¼ ounce (7 g) dried lavender flowers ¼ cup (60 ml) evening primrose oil ¼ cup (54 g) coconut oil 1 cup (200 g) raw sugar 10 drops tea tree essential oil 10 drops chamomile essential oil	YIELD: 1 cup (235 ml) Preheat oven to 170°F (77°C). Place lavender flowers in a shallow glass baking dish and pour oils over them. Bake for 4 hours. Strain. Add sugar and essential oils. Mix together and transfer to a storage container. I prefer to use this in the shower with a little moisture. Apply small amounts gently in a circular motion; rinse well.

LONGEVITY

My personality lives in the depths of emotion and cravings for connection. Seeing people and experiences beyond the surface is something I'm accustomed to. I feel what others feel, and I see what others often don't want to see. This has proven to be both a blessing and, at times, excruciatingly frustrating. But it has also repeatedly reminded me of how much I love being alive. This always ties into my longing to live forever, not because I'm afraid to pass on but because I love being human, in the life I live. And it isn't because my life is perfect and without troubles. Believe you me, I've had to learn from mistakes over and over. It is simply the joy of seeing the trees, smelling the flowers, and holding the people I love.

I can't promise you'll live to be one hundred, but some of these formulas are touted to help you get there.

BRAIN HEALTH TINCTURE

Keeping our brain active is important as we age. This formula helps ensure that blood flow and oxygenation are staying active as well.

1½ teaspoons (8 ml) sage tincture	**YIELD:** 1 ounce (28 ml)
1½ teaspoons (8 ml) rosemary tincture	Combine all ingredients in a 1-ounce
1½ teaspoons (8 ml) ginkgo tincture	(28 ml) amber dropper bottle.
1 teaspoon (5 ml) turmeric tincture	Take 1 dropperful 2 to 3 times per day.
¼ teaspoon (1 ml) cayenne tincture	

LONG LIFE ELIXIR

Elixirs are often touted as longevity potions, providing stamina and vigor to the weak. This recipe has been around the block, and it definitely produces an extra beat in your step.

1 ounce (28 g) dried Ashwagandha root	**YIELD:** 1 quart (946 ml)
½ ounce (14 g) dried Damiana leaf	Soak herbs in brandy for 3 to 4 weeks.
1 ounce (28 g) dried American ginseng root	Strain. Transfer to a storage container.
½ ounce (14 g) dried Ginkgo leaf	Drink 1 ounce (28 ml) 3 to 4 times per
1 ounce (28 g) dried Licorice root	week, or as needed. Alternatively, you can
½ ounce (15 g) cinnamon chips	take 1 to 2 dropperfuls each day.
1 quart (946 ml) brandy	

PEACE OF MIND CORDIAL

Cordials have been recorded in herbal history for centuries. *Cordial* literally means "warm and friendly" or "for the heart," with this healing drink applying both. It's a warm and friendly drink that benefits the heart. When the heart is at peace, you are at peace. Consider making this in the fall to have on hand for the winter months.

1 bottle of red table wine

1 ounce (28 g) dried hawthorn berry

1 ounce (28 g) dried burdock root

½ ounce (14 g) dried astragalus root

½ ounce (14 g) dried holy basil leaf

¼ ounce (7 g) dried dong quai root

1 ounce (28 g) fresh ginger root

¼ ounce (7.5 g) cinnamon chips

5 whole cloves

Dried fruit, such as apricots (optional)

YIELD: Varies depending on fruit

Pour the wine into a gallon (3.7 L) glass jar and add the remaining ingredients. Let infuse for 3 to 4 weeks in a cool, dark place; be sure to shake the mixture from time to time. After the infusion time has passed, strain out the herbs and then strain again using fine mesh cloth to remove all particulates. Store in a pretty decanter bottle and drink 1-ounce (28 ml) doses with a friend while sitting next to the fire and telling secret stories of winters past.

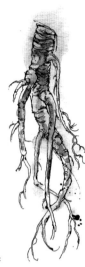

Dong Quai

VARIATION: STRONG AND STEADY TINCTURE

For an overall longevity tonic, you can't go wrong with the following herbal blend. It supports youthfulness, immune system health, and stamina health. It can be made into a tincture, a tea, or placed in a capsule.

1 part fo-ti

1 part ashwagandha

1 part hawthorn flowers

YIELD: Varies, depending on form

Combine equal parts and prepare as normal, depending if you would like a tincture, a tea, or a capsule. If you prefer a tea, you can add a pinch of any of the following flavor combinations.

Licorice and ginger

Mint and honey

Lemongrass and clove

JOINT RESCUE

Our body, despite our best efforts, does begin to break down over the years. That doesn't mean everything has to be explained by "It's just what happens, I'm getting old!" More and more care is necessary as we age; it is simply cause and effect. This formula will help you get out of bed a little easier in the morning by reducing stiffness and sore joints.

½ ounce (14 g) turmeric powder	**YIELD**: 200 capsules
½ ounce (14 g) devil's claw powder	Combine all powders in a bowl. Use
½ ounce (14 g) boswellia powder	mixture to fill empty vegetable capsules.
½ ounce (14 g) ginger powder	Take 2 capsules twice daily
	for maintenance.

SLEEP

Anyone who has stayed up late recently has most likely seen the effects on their face. Enough sleep is one of the best ways to not only stay healthy but also to keep your skin glowing. My tips?

- Try to get eight to nine hours of sleep each night.
- Try to go to bed before 11 p.m. in order to follow natural circadian rhythms.
- Stop all technologic activities thirty minutes before bedtime.
- Have a cup of tea that promotes sleep and relaxation one hour before bedtime.
- Take Sleep Tincture at bedtime (see page 204).

SLEEP TEA

A cup of calming herbs an hour before bedtime should bring the sandman knocking at your bedroom door.

1 ounce (28 g) dried hawthorn berry	**YIELD**: 4 ounces (112 g)
½ ounce (14 g) dried skullcap leaf	Combine all herbs; store in a glass jar
½ ounce (14 g) dried chamomile flower	until needed. Make by the cup: Steep 1 to
1 tablespoon (3 g) dried hops	2 teaspoons (1.5 to 3 g) per 10 ounces
1 ounce (28 g) dried peppermint leaf	(280 ml) of boiling water, covered, for
	8 to 10 minutes.

SLEEP TINCTURE

Sometimes you just need a little help falling asleep. Whether you are sick or stressed, this blend is sure to nudge you into the sleep zone. It's not to be used as treatment for chronic insomnia.

4 teaspoons (20 ml) hops tincture	YIELD: 1 ounce (28 ml)
2 teaspoons (10 ml) California poppy tincture	Combine all ingredients in a 2-ounce (60 ml)
2 teaspoons (10 ml) hawthorn berry tincture	amber dropper bottle. Take 1 to 2 dropperfuls as needed.

FIRST AID 101

A basic herbal first-aid kit is a very handy thing. Whether you need something for yourself, a family member, or a friend, being able to go to the cabinet and quickly treat the situation you're presented with is both helpful and rewarding. Add to it:

Salve for cuts, burns, scrapes

Anti-itch salve

Earache oil

Poison oak/ivy liniment

Cold and flu tea and capsules

Stomachache essential oil blend

Antidiarrhea solutions

Sore throat spray

Cough syrup

Mouth healing rinse

Muscle liniment

Sleep Tincture

Calming tea

Various adhesive bandages

BASIC FIRST-AID SALVE

This all-purpose salve can be used for kitchen burns, sunburns, bug bites, cuts, and scrapes. When in doubt, I put this on. The great thing about a salve is that it forms a natural bandage over the wound, keeping it protected.

½ ounce (14 g) calendula flower	YIELD: 8 ounces (235 ml)
¼ ounce (7 g) lavender flower	Preheat oven to 170°F (77°C). Place herbs in a shallow
¼ ounce (7 g) comfrey leaf	baking dish and pour olive oil over them. Give a little
1 cup (235 ml) olive oil	stir. Bake for 4 hours. Strain. Pour into a saucepan and
1 ounce (28 g) beeswax	turn to low. Add beeswax and stir until melted. Let cool
40 drops lavender essential oil	for a couple of minutes and add essential oil. Pour into a lidded storage container or containers. Let cool completely before closing the container.

ANTI-ITCH SALVE

My sweet daughter Cordelia cannot help but scratch a mosquito bite. I get it; the itch is maddening, and the instant gratification is so good when you do scratch. But as we all know, once a bite is scratched, it itches forever. This salve was created for her.

½ ounce (14 g) dried chaparral leaf

½ ounce (14 g) black walnut hull

½ ounce (14 g) dried juniper berry

¼ ounce (7 g) dried calendula flower

¼ ounce (7 g) whole cloves

1½ cups (355 ml) olive oil

1 to 2 ounces (28 to 56 g) beeswax, depending on preferred consistency

40 drops peppermint essential oil

YIELD: 10 ounces (285 ml)

Preheat oven to 170°F (77°C). Place herbs in a shallow baking dish and pour olive oil over them. Give a little stir. Bake for 4 hours. Strain. Pour into a saucepan and turn to low. Add 1 to 2 ounces (28 to 56 g) of beeswax and stir until melted. Let cool for a couple of minutes and add essential oil. Pour into a storage container or containers. Let cool completely before closing the container.

EARACHE OIL

This one can be a lifesaver, especially for children. The important piece regarding this formula is that it must be made in summer, when mullein flowers are in bloom.

Mullein flowers

Olive oil

10 cloves garlic

YIELD: Varies, depending on the freshness of the flowers

When the fresh mullein flowers are opening early in the morning, collect them in a pint (473 ml) jar. Fill up the jar and then pour olive oil over them until it reaches the top. Close the jar well and give it a good shake. Set the jar where it will receive sun all day long. While it's sitting during the day, you can take the lid off and drape a kitchen towel over the jar to allow water from the fresh flowers an opportunity to evaporate. Each day, close the jar up and give it another good shake. Allow to sun soak for 2 to 3 weeks; strain. Transfer to a clean, sterile container, preferably with a dropper.

While the mullein is sun soaking, create a second oil—a garlic oil. Simply place 10 open garlic cloves in 1 cup (235 ml) of olive oil and let them steep for 3 to 4 weeks. Strain and transfer to a separate container.

Into a 2-ounce (60 ml) dropper bottle, pour 4 teaspoons (20 ml) of the mullein flower oil and 2 teaspoons (10 ml) of the garlic oil. Close the bottle and shake. You now have ready-to-use earache oil. Place

(continued)

2 to 3 drops of oil in each ear at the first sign of ear infection or pain, 2 to 3 times per day. Massage all around ear after application.

I like to keep the oils separate. That way I can use them for other things should I desire.

POISON OAK/IVY LINIMENT

When poison oak strikes, you want to be prepared. Avoid all oil-based products when treating these rashes, as they will spread the plant oils that are causing the inflammation. Wash the affected area with soap and tepid water 3 to 4 times per day. Change your bed sheets and clothes each day, and don't shower in hot water. These steps, combined with the topical application of the following formula, should help move the rash along.

1 ounce (28 g) dried white oak bark	**YIELD:** 1 pint (473 ml)
1 ounce (28 g) dried mugwort leaf	Soak all herbs in rubbing alcohol for 3 to 4 weeks.
1 ounce (28 g) dried plantain leaf	Strain and transfer to a storage container. Label and
1 pint (473 ml) rubbing alcohol	have cotton balls nearby for when it's needed.

COLD AND FLU CAPSULES

Take 2 capsules at the first sign of sniffles or body aches.

¼ ounce (7 g) echinacea powder	**YIELD:** Varies
¼ ounce (7 g) boneset powder	Combine all powders in a bowl. Use the mixture to
¼ ounce (7 g) yarrow powder	fill at least 20 empty vegetable capsules to have on
¼ ounce (7 g) goldenseal powder	hand when needed.

HEAD COLD TEA

Opening up the nasal passageways when you have a head cold can quickly improve your quality of existence. Smelling the volatile peppermint oils from the cup are a great secondary treatment when you drink it.

1 ounce (28 g) dried peppermint	**YIELD:** 3 ounces (84 g)
1 ounce (28 g) dried chamomile	Combine all herbs; store in an airtight container until
½ ounce (14 g) dried elderflower	needed. To make a cup of tea, steep 2 teaspoons
½ ounce (14 g) dried yarrow flower	(3 g) of tea in a cup of boiling water, covered, for
¼ ounce (7 g) dried ginger root	8 to 10 minutes.

Stomach Flu

Have charcoal capsules and castor oil packs on hand for support. Take two charcoal capsules as soon as you are able to keep something down, and apply a castor oil pack each day you aren't feeling well. See page 102 for a complete guide on how to use a castor oil pack.

STOMACHACHE ESSENTIAL OIL BLEND

This is one of my go-tos for any little (or big) one who reports an ache in the belly.

40 drops fennel essential oil

20 drops lavender essential oil

20 drops catnip essential oil

3 ounces (45 ml) sweet apricot oil

1 ounce (28 ml) castor oil

YIELD: 4 ounces (120 ml)

Combine all oils and store in a 4-ounce (60 ml) amber bottle. Rub 1 to 2 teaspoons (5 to 10 ml) all over the abdomen in gentle circular motions. Add a hot water bottle on top afterward, if desired.

ANTIDIARRHEA TINCTURE

Sometimes it just needs to stop. This tincture can help to slow down the urgency of diarrhea.

2 teaspoons (10 ml) Oregon grape root tincture

1 teaspoon (5 ml) red raspberry leaf tincture

1 teaspoon (5 ml) agrimony leaf

1 teaspoon (5 ml) chamomile flower tincture

1 teaspoon (5 ml) barberry tincture

YIELD: 1 ounce (28 ml)

Combine all ingredients in a 1-ounce (28 ml) dropper bottle. Take 2 dropperfuls 4 to 6 times per day or until diarrhea lessens. See your medical practitioner if there's no change after 24 hours.

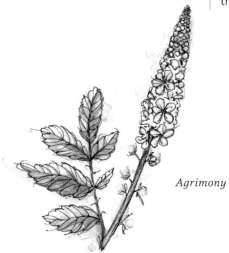

Agrimony

Activated Charcoal Powder for Diarrhea

Activated charcoal powder and capsules are used to treat adults, children, and infants for acute diarrhea. Mervyn G. Hardinge, M.D., Dr. P.H., Ph.D., the founding dean of the School of Public Health at Loma Linda University, places charcoal under the heading of "harmless" in his most recent book, *Drugs, Herbs, & Natural Remedies*. Used to bind toxins and poisons that have entered the body, activated charcoal can safely help those struggling from active diarrhea discomforts.

DOSAGES: **Adults:** 2 to 4 capsules every 4 hours or until diarrhea subsides

Children: 1 to 2 capsules every 4 hours or until diarrhea subsides

Infants: 1 capsule opened and added to softened food every 6 hours or until diarrhea subsides

SORE THROAT SPRAY

This is another good one to have ready to go. Sore throats seem to come out of nowhere, so make this at the beginning of winter to have on hand.

1 ounce (28 g) dried echinacea root	YIELD: 2 cups (475 ml)
1 ounce (28 g) dried elderberries	Place herbs in a pint (473 ml) jar and pour ¼ cup
½ ounce (14 g) dried sage leaf	(60 ml) of boiling water over them. Close jar and let
½ ounce (14 g) dried thyme leaf	steep for 1 hour. Add vodka and vegetable glycerin.
¼ ounce (7 g) dried peppermint leaf	Close again and give a good shake. Let soak for
¼ cup (60 ml) vodka	3 weeks, shaking every day. Strain and transfer into
½ cup (120 ml) vegetable glycerin	one big container or into multiple 2-ounce (60 ml)
20 drops lemon essential oil	bottles with spray tops. I like to have one at home,
5 drops clove essential oil	one at work, one in the car, etc. Add essential oils
	to each bottle; close, shake to blend, and label.
	Use 1 to 2 sprays as needed for sore throat, 4 to
	6 times per day.

COUGH SYRUP

Syrups in general are the easiest way to get anyone to take herbal medicine, mainly because they are sugar or honey based. For years, I used honey as my syrup base, but recently I've returned to pure cane sugar because I've found more and more honey to be adulterated—and it's expensive. Sugar also has a longer preservation factor; if I'm making a year's batch at a time, I like to ensure it won't ferment on me. There is a lot of debate on the use of sugar in herbal products, but I find it to work well and be cost-effective, with few side effects or worsening of symptoms.

1 ounce (28 g) dried licorice root

1 ounce (28 g) dried marshmallow root

1 ounce (28 g) dried wild cherry bark

½ ounce (14 g) dried horehound leaf

½ ounce (14 g) dried mullein leaf

½ ounce (14 g) dried coltsfoot leaf

Sugar or honey

YIELD: 2 cups (475 ml)

Place the first 3 ingredients in a large stockpot or Dutch oven. Pour 6 cups (1.4 L) of water over them. Cover and bring to a boil over high heat.

Give a quick stir, cover, and simmer over low heat for 10 minutes. Add the next 3 ingredients, give another quick stir, cover, and let simmer for another 5 minutes. Then turn off the heat and let steep for 2 hours.

Strain and measure the total liquid. Pour liquid back into the now-clean pot and add sugar or honey in an amount equal to one-half the volume of the existing brew.

A 2:1 herb-to-sugar ratio means that if you have 4 cups (950 ml) of brew after straining, you add 2 cups sugar (200 g) or honey (680 g). Some people prefer sweeter syrup and use a 1:1 ratio, so follow your preference.

Gently heat mixture if needed to dissolve sugar thoroughly. Allow to completely cool; bottle up and label for future use.

MOUTH RINSE EXTRACT

This is one I like to have on hand because canker sores, sore teeth, and sore gums can arise without warning. The following is made with herbal tinctures, yet used like a mouthwash.

1 tablespoon (15 ml) white willow bark tincture

1 teaspoon (5 ml) lemon balm leaf tincture

1 teaspoon (5 ml) clove, whole tincture

1 teaspoon (5 ml) white oak bark tincture

5 drops clove essential oil (or peppermint or cinnamon)

YIELD: 1 ounce (28 ml)

Combine all ingredients in a 1-ounce (28 ml) amber dropper bottle. Use daily as a preventative or daily for 3 months as treatment. Put 1 to 2 dropperfuls in 1 ounce (28 ml) of warm water. Rinse for 1 minute; spit out.

MUSCLE LINIMENT

For the daily aches and pains of life, it's good to have something to provide temporary relief. A liniment provides heat and cooling at the same time.

1 tablespoon (2.5 g) peppermint leaf

1 tablespoon (2 g) eucalyptus leaf

1 tablespoon (2 g) St. John's wort herb

1 tablespoon (15 g) ginkgo leaf

1 tablespoon (6 g) turmeric root

1 tablespoon (6 g) ginger root

1 teaspoon (4 g) menthol crystals

1 cup (235 ml) witch hazel extract, plus more to top off jar if necessary

YIELD: 1 pint (473 ml)

Combine all ingredients in a pint (473 ml) jar. Top it off with witch hazel extract if needed. Cover and shake. Let steep for 4 weeks, shaking the jar daily. Strain and transfer to a storage container; I prefer a spray-top bottle for easy application.

Spray 2 to 4 times on aching areas as needed. Ideally, have someone else massage the liniment in for deeper application.

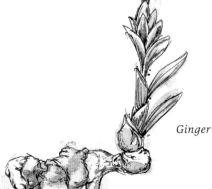

Ginger

CALMING TEA

Every household should have this tea available. Whether it is for you or someone else, it will promote calmness from the first sip. Make a batch of the following or create your own. Label it clearly and leave it where everyone can see it. Having it accessible allows anyone to ask for a cup and moment of calm.

1 ounce (28 g) dried skullcap

1 ounce (28 g) dried agrimony

2 ounces (56 g) dried chamomile

1 ounce (28 g) dried passionflower

1 ounce (28 g) dried lemongrass

3 ounces (84 g) dried peppermint

YIELD: 9 ounces (252 g)
Combine all herbs; store in a clear mason jar for everyone to see. Use 1 to 2 teaspoons (1.5 to 3 g) per 1 cup (235 ml) of water to make tea as needed.

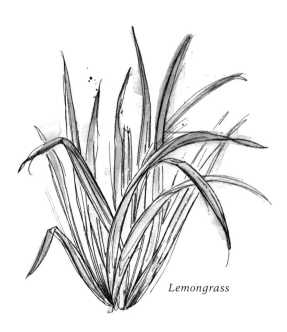

Lemongrass

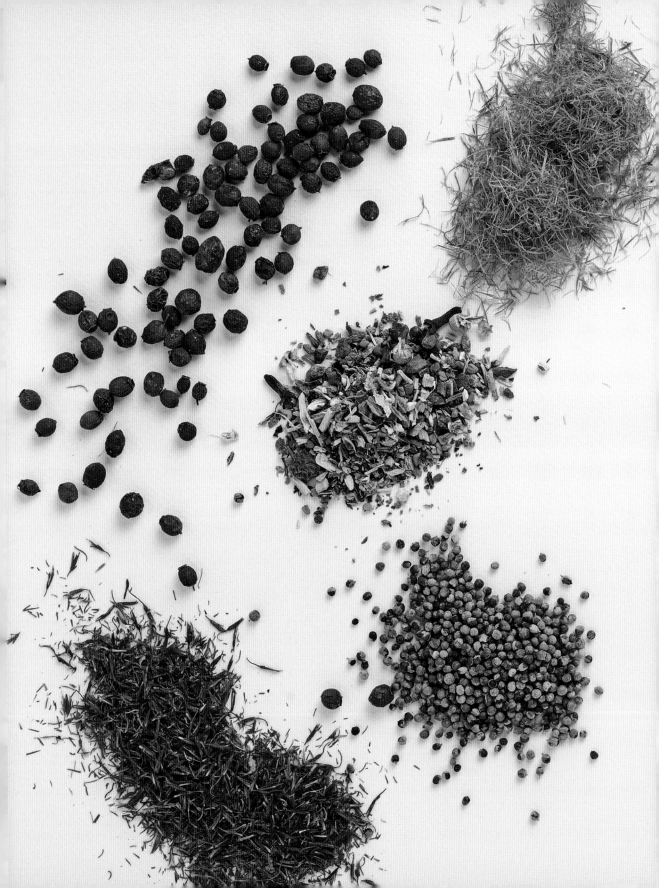

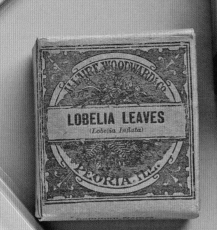

CHAPTER 7

———

Support

THESE DAYS, DISORDERS of the thyroid, adrenal glands, heart, liver, and bladder seem to be all too common. Whether the problems are genetically based or acquired through modern living, it has become necessary to care for all areas of our body. Because prevention is key, I've included the following information and recipes to offer support for these systems.

LIVER HEALTH

The liver is the main organ responsible for hormone production and detoxification for the entire body. This is no small task. This organ is so valuable that the body was designed to regenerate it if needed. You can lose up to 70 percent of your liver and it will work its way to full regeneration if given the chance. It is truly one of the most fascinating organs of our body.

As we go through life, we place many demands on our liver. With the development of genetically modified organisms (GMOs), synthetic medications, food preservatives, and environmental toxins, our modern livers are working overtime. In Chinese medicine, the liver is considered the general of the body; its job is to plan, organize, and direct all bodily functions. Chinese medicine also considers the liver the house of all emotion. It states that if the liver is healthy and well, emotions will be appropriate and even. But if the liver is burdened, its energy can slow down, leading to a rise in imbalanced emotions such as depression, frustration, and repressed anger. Therefore, supporting the liver can only improve physical and emotional well-being. This leads to hormonal balance, decreased stress, and a body free of waste.

When to use the following recipes? If you are living a relatively healthy lifestyle, my suggestion is to spend one month each year devoted to a different body system. For example, every March I focus on my liver. I drink the Liver Love Tea (see right) each day and put daily castor oil packs on my abdomen. The castor oil supports the liver's detoxification efforts. Another option is to simply rotate in your supportive teas, capsules, tinctures, and topical treatments throughout the year.

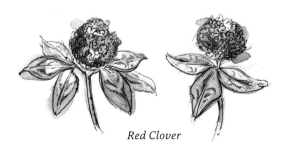

Red Clover

LIVER LOVE TEA

This blend supports overall function of the liver and can be used regularly as a liver tonic.

1 ounce (28 g) dried burdock root	YIELD: 7 ounces (196 g)
1 ounce (28 g) dried dandelion root	Combine all ingredients; store in a glass
1 ounce (28 g) dried red clover	jar. Make by the cup or make medicinally
1 ounce (28 g) dried white oak bark	(page 245) with 5 tablespoons (22 g)
1 ounce (28 g) dried milk thistle seeds	in a quart (1 liter) of almost boiling water;
2 ounces (56 g) dried spearmint leaf or ½ ounce (14 g) each ginger root, cinnamon bark, and licorice root, depending on your flavor preference	let steep overnight.

LIVER TONE AND BLOOD BUILDING TINCTURE

This is a wonderfully nourishing mixture of herbs for the liver that support function and health of the hepatocytes.

2 tablespoons (30 ml) bupleurum tincture	YIELD: 4 ounces (120 ml)
2 tablespoons (30 ml) milk thistle seed tincture	Combine all ingredients in a 4-ounce
2 tablespoons (30 ml) dandelion root tincture	(120 ml) amber dropper bottle. Take
1 tablespoon (15 ml) dong quai tincture	1 dropperful 3 times per day as desired;
1 tablespoon (15 ml) nettle leaf tincture	for a more tonifying effect, take
	consistently for 3 to 6 weeks.

INFUSED CASTOR OIL PACK FOR THE LIVER

If you've ever seen a naturopathic physician, you are probably quite familiar with a castor oil pack. Nature cure at its best is clearly demonstrated with this therapy. By utilizing the healing and anti-inflammatory agents of the castor plant, you can greatly support the liver in improved function and health.

18 ounces (500 ml) castor oil	YIELD: 18 ounces (500 ml)
4 ounces (120 ml) olive oil	Combine all ingredients in a slow cooker
½ ounce (14 g) dried red clover leaf	and cook on low for 1 week to infuse.
½ ounce (14 g) dried yellow dock root	Store in a glass jar in a cool dark place.
½ ounce (14 g) dried artichoke leaf	Strain and apply daily to abdomen with
½ ounce (14 g) dried burdock root	gentle heat for 30 to 45 minutes.

SKIN GLOW TINCTURE

Skin health is often a reflection of liver health. When the liver is backed up processing waste, the skin picks up the slack and starts to purge through our outer layers. This tincture works to support both the liver detoxification pathways and the health of the skin.

3 tablespoons (40 ml) dandelion root tincture	YIELD: 4 ounces (120 ml)
2 tablespoons (30 ml) marshmallow root tincture	Combine all ingredients in a 4-ounce
4 teaspoons (20 ml) saw palmetto berry tincture	(120 ml) amber dropper bottle.
4 teaspoons (20 ml) wild yam root tincture	Take 1 dropperful 3 times per day
2 teaspoons (10 ml) echinacea root tincture	for 4 to 6 weeks.

BASIC BALANCE: HORMONE LIVER SUPPORT TINCTURE

Get to the root of the imbalance by encouraging liver hormonal health.

2 tablespoons (30 ml) bupleurum root tincture	YIELD: 4 ounces (120 ml)
2 tablespoons (30 ml) dandelion root tincture	Combine all ingredients in a 4-ounce
1 tablespoon (15 ml) dong quai root tincture	(120 ml) amber dropper bottle.
1 tablespoon (15 ml) yellow dock root tincture	Take 1 dropperful 3 times per day
1 tablespoon (15 ml) wild yam room tincture	for 8 to 12 weeks.
1 tablespoon (15 ml) black cohosh root tincture	

DIGESTIVE SUPPORT

Babies poop and we say, "Oh! You pooped! Good job!" like they've just learned to walk or talk. The function is often exclaimed over and praised joyfully, and the babies feel so proud that they've done this miraculous thing. As we age, this simple eliminatory function can become challenged and troublesome. Sometimes it becomes so difficult that when you do finally have a successful bowel movement, you almost want to jump up and down and pat yourself on the back. When and how did our digestive systems get so off track? IBS (irritable bowel syndrome), Crohn's disease, leaky gut, and so on are twenty-first-century problems, and they are almost now considered mainstream. I have a few theories as to why that is, but what I do know is that when I educate my patients on how to get back to the basics of digestion, things improve.

Dr. JJ's tips for a healthy digestion:

- Eat at roughly the same time every day.
- Give your body adequate time to recognize that it's eating time. You do this by looking at and smelling food as you prepare it. This turns on the digestive function before you begin eating so that the system can be prepared and ready for when food arrives in the stomach. Try this instead of multitasking, with work one minute and shoving a burrito down your throat the next. Eating in this fashion often catches the body off guard and completely unprepared to digest food.
- Use herbs before and after eating to aid the elimination process. Bitters are a great choice; they can increase digestion success and decrease digestion upset.

HEARTBURN SUPPORT CAPSULES

Although it is always best to identify the cause of heartburn, these capsules will soothe the burn and relieve the suffering in the moment.

1 ounce (28 g) gentian root powder	**YIELD:** 100 capsules
½ ounce (14 g) skullcap leaf powder	Combine all ingredients in a bowl. Use the
½ ounce (14 g) ginger root powder	mixture to fill empty vegetable capsules. Take 2 capsules with every meal.

AFTER DINNER SPOT OF TEA

Drink this tea to encourage healthy digestion and ease of the digestive process.

1 ounce (28 g) dried gentian root	**YIELD:** 3 ounces (84 g)
1 ounce (28 g) dried chamomile flowers	Combine all ingredients; store in a glass
½ ounce (14 g) dried fennel seed	jar. Put on the kettle as you are clearing
¼ ounce (7 g) dried anise seed	the table. Use 1 to 2 teaspoons (1.5 to 3 g) per cup (235 ml) hot water. Let steep 10 minutes; strain before drinking.

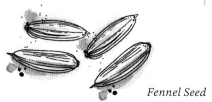

Fennel Seed

OVERINDULGENCE TINCTURE

We all do it. But you don't have to suffer from celebrating, whether that means overeating or indulging in the types of foods—fatty or rich, for example—that don't make your body feel good.

2 tablespoons (30 ml) fenugreek seed tincture

2 tablespoons (30 ml) fennel seed tincture

4 teaspoons (20 ml) gentian tincture

4 teaspoons (20 ml) catnip tincture

2 teaspoons (10 ml) marshmallow root tincture

2 teaspoons (10 ml) licorice root tincture

YIELD: 4 ounces (120 ml)

Combine all ingredients in a 4-ounce (120 ml) amber dropper bottle. Take 2 to 3 dropperfuls at the first sign of overeating. Take 2 more dropperfuls 30 minutes later.

INTESTINAL REPAIR TEA

Long-term inflammation due to poor dietary choices and stress can damage the intestinal track. This blend works hard to heal it. By nourishing and supporting the structure of the intestines, your energy will increase and digestive management get back on track.

2 ounces (56 g) dried cranesbill root

1 ounce (28 g) dried marshmallow root

½ ounce (14 g) dried goldenseal root

½ ounce (14 g) dried plantain leaf

½ to 1 ounce (14 to 28 g) dried ginger root

½ ounce (14 g) dried fennel seed, optional

YIELD: 5 ounces (140 g)

Combine all ingredients; store in a glass jar. To make a cup of tea, simmer 1 to 2 teaspoons (1.5 to 3 g) per 1 cup (235 ml) of hot water, covered, over low heat. After 10 minutes, turn off heat and add 1 teaspoon (1.5 g) more of the blend. Let steep 10 minutes. Drink 2 to 3 cups per day for 4 to 6 weeks.

VARIATION: INTESTINAL REPAIR TINCTURE

If you'd prefer drops versus a tea, here is the above recipe as a tincture.

3 tablespoons (40 ml) cranesbill root tincture

4 teaspoons (20 ml) marshmallow root tincture

4 teaspoons (20 ml) goldenseal root tincture

4 teaspoons (20 ml) plantain leaf tincture

2 teaspoons (10 ml) ginger root tincture

2 teaspoons (10 ml) fennel seed tincture

YIELD: 4 ounces (120 ml)

Combine all ingredients in a 4-ounce (120 ml) amber dropper bottle. Take 1 dropperful 3 times per day for 4 to 6 weeks.

DIARRHEA RELIEF TEA

It's never a good day when you are suffering from diarrhea. Do yourself a favor and be proactive in your care.

Note: Chronic diarrhea should be addressed by seeking professional care.

1 ounce (28 g) dried Cranesbill root

1 ounce (28 g) dried Oregon grape

½ ounce (14 g) dried Echinacea

½ ounce (14 g) dried Agrimony

½ ounce (14 g) dried Catnip

1 ounce (28 g) dried lemongrass

YIELD: 4 ounces (112 g)

Combine all ingredients; store in a glass jar. Simmer 1 to 2 teaspoons (1.5 to 3 g) per 1 cup (235 ml) of hot water, covered, over low heat. After 10 minutes, turn off heat and add 1 teaspoon (1.5 g) more of the blend. Let steep 10 minutes. Drink 1 to 3 cups as needed throughout the day.

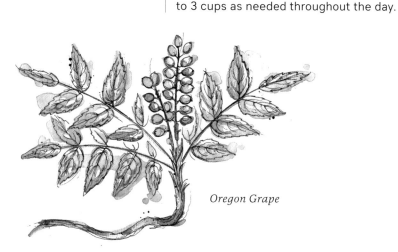

Oregon Grape

DIGESTION SPECIFIC CASTOR OIL PACK

This treatment is meant to slow down the evacuation of the bowels and alleviate inflammation. Apply this castor oil pack at the first sign of loose stool.

18 ounces (500 ml) castor oil

4 ounces (120 ml) olive oil

2 ounces (56 g) dried fennel seed

1 ounce (28 g) dried agrimony leaf

½ ounce (14 g) dried catnip

½ ounce (14 g) dried chamomile flower

YIELD: 1 castor oil pack

Place all ingredients in a slow cooker; heat on low for 1 week to infuse. Strain and store in a glass jar until needed. Apply daily to abdomen with gentle heat for 30 to 45 minutes.

CONSTIPATION CANDY

This is a great recipe that I've passed along many times over. Eating 1 to 2 of these candies a day can encourage relief of the bowel without an emergency trip to the bathroom.

1 ounce (28 g) slippery elm powder	YIELD: 12 candy balls
1 ounce (28 g) dried senna leaf	Mix all ingredients together thoroughly; form into 1-inch (3 cm) balls. Store in an airtight container in the refrigerator for up to 2 weeks.
1 ounce (28 g) dried marshmallow root	
½ cup (120 ml) aloe vera juice	
¼ cup (21.5 g) cacao powder	
½ cup (130 g) nut butter of choice (optional)	
Honey to achieve desired consistency	

BEDTIME TEA FOR MORNING RELIEF

This blend is considered gently laxative in nature, not purgative. That means it works slowly and on a gentler plane then a purgative. Purgatives create intense spasms to clear the bowel out, often leading to a run to the bathroom when it strikes. Take before bed to help the morning go smooth.

2 ounces (56 g) dried gentian root	YIELD: 4 ounces (112 g)
1 ounce (28 g) dried marshmallow root	Combine all ingredients; store in a glass jar. When needed, steep 1 to 2 teaspoons (1.5 to 3 g) per 1 cup (235 ml) of hot water for 10 minutes.
½ ounce (14 g) dried licorice root	
½ ounce (14 g) dried senna leaf	

GET THOSE JUICES FLOWING!

This is an effective bitters tincture for pre- and post meals. Bitters is one of the best ways to kick off proper digestion.

2 tablespoonss (30 ml) orange peel tincture	YIELD: 4 ounces (120 ml)
1½ tablespoons (25 ml) gentian tincture	Combine all ingredients in a 2-ounce (60 ml) amber dropper bottle. Take 1 to 2 dropperfuls 10 minutes before and after meals.
1½ tablespoons (25 ml) angelica tincture	
1½ tablespoons (25 ml) fennel seed tincture	
4 teaspoons (20 ml) ginger tincture	

BREAST HEALTH

Breasts. If only we could reshape our society's view of this female body part. Highly sexualized, the breasts are undervalued and highly criticized in both their function and appearance. They come in all shapes and sizes, and though loving what we are born with is necessary, it is not taught. Often breasts can be viewed as cumbersome or embarrassing, depending on how the community we surround ourselves with views them. Exquisitely feminine, they are a universal symbol of the female and mother. Although their most obvious job is to create and secrete breast milk for offspring, they also respond to sexual stimulation and estrogen and progesterone through receptor sites in the breast tissue. This is most often seen around the menstrual cycle, as breast tissue can swell and become tender.

As with any aspect of the lymphatic system (the breasts include an extensive amount of lymphatic tissue), proper circulation is vital to health. Stagnation of surrounding fluid and consumption of lymph congestive substances (like coffee, unfortunately) can result in breast tissue changes. Yes, giving up that regular coffee habit can make a big difference, resulting in smoother breast tissue, but so can regular breast massage. Even better, using an herbal lymphatic breast oil will move and break up fibrotic tissue, which feels like lumps in the breast. Herbs such as poke root, cleavers, and even dandelion root all support breast health.

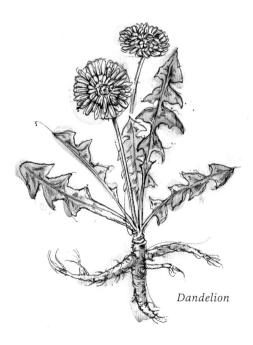

Dandelion

BREAST HEALTH MASSAGE OIL

This blend focuses on reducing fibrotic breast tissue and improving lymphatic flow through the breasts.

1 ounce (28 g) dried poke root

½ ounce (14 g) dried chamomile flower

½ ounce (14 g) dried dandelion root

1½ cups (355 ml) olive oil

20 drops grapefruit essential oil

10 drops rosemary essential oil

YIELD: 1 to 2 ounces (29 to 60 ml)

Preheat oven to 170°F (77°C). Place herbs in a glass baking dish and pour olive oil over them. Bake for 4 hours. Strain and transfer to a 1- or 2-ounce (29 or 60 ml) amber bottle. Add essential oils. Use this oil a few times a week in the shower; rub 1 to 2 teaspoons (5 to 10 ml) on each breast and massage in a slow circular motion for a couple minutes.

NIPPLE HEALTH

Make a mask for your nipple to encourage healthy glow and texture to this unique skin.

1 ounce (28 g) powdered calendula flowers

1 ounce (28 g) powdered rose petals

½ ounce (14 g) powered comfrey leaf

½ ounce (14 g) powdered elderberry flowers

½ ounce (14 g) French green clay

YIELD: 4 ounces (98 g)

Mix all ingredients together; store in a glass jar. For treatment, place 1 to 3 tablespoons (15 to 45 g) of the blend in a bowl. Add just enough hot water to make a spreadable paste; apply to both nipples. Be sure to completely cover the entire areola. Let sit for 10 to 15 minutes with a warm towel covering the breasts. Wash gently with warm water afterward and apply Day-to-Day Breast Oil.

DAY-TO-DAY BREAST OIL

Our breasts, like any body part, need to be nourished and touched regularly. Recognizing your breasts is important—it mobilizes energy and reduces stagnation. Take a moment and visualize energy moving all throughout your body, including your breasts. Then apply this daily breast oil after each shower. Learn and love your breast terrain.

4 ounces (120 ml) jojoba oil

40 drops neroli essential oil

5 drops vetiver essential oil

YIELD: 4 ounces (120 ml)

Place all ingredients in a 4-ounce (120 ml) amber bottle with a therapeutic pump. Use 1 to 2 pumps per breast each day.

STRESS ATTACKS

Stress attacks are moments when you feel anxiety, anxiousness, panic, insomnia, adrenalized, explosive, or knocked out from fatigue. As we move through life, our ability to compensate physically, mentally, and emotionally can be challenged. If stress is on auto repeat in our lives, we begin to get worse and worse at handling the physical and emotional symptoms that arise as a result. Many of my young patients don't know how to recognize stress in their lives. Once we discuss the above symptoms, they often realize they've been living with it for a while. What I see most commonly in my practice is stress caused by the following:

- Overworking
- Taking on too much
- Being overly involved in too many activities
- Lack of exercise or some other sort of healthy release
- Relationship stress: intimate, familial, or professional
- Lack of resources: home, money, food
- Situational stress: midterms, a project deadline, a relationship ending

If any one of these situations is occurring, the central nervous system and the adrenal glands step up to the plate to support you. The problem is, after repetitive stress "attacks," the body declines in its ability to calm everything back down. It's like your favorite slippers. After putting them on and off, over and over, they wear out.

Our adrenal glands particularly are affected by stress. They support the release of cortisol, the stress hormone. Stress can take the form of decreased blood sugar, pain, inflammation, or emotional upset. When any of these occur, we release cortisol to "handle" the situation. The problem is that when we don't address our body's physical and emotional needs appropriately, we sail into cortisol autopilot zone, which dumps cortisol right and left, thinking that is what is best. Learning to regulate our adrenals takes practice, support, and nourishment.

If you are experiencing any stress symptoms, consider the recipes below to nourish and support both the central nervous system and the adrenal glands. Meanwhile, here are some basic tips for adrenal nourishment.

1. Wake up and go to bed at approximately the same time each day to regulate circadian and hormonal patterns.
2. Eat within an hour of the same time each day to better regulate blood sugar.

3. Find a daily outlet of release: a ritual cup of tea, a meditation, exercise, etc.

4. If you have chronic pain or inflammation, treat it with herbs, diet, or body treatments such as massage or physical therapy, and don't repeat the stressors that cause it to continue.

5. Make a list of your daily stressors. Include everything, no matter how big or how small, even if you think there is nothing you can do about it. Write them all down. Choose one at a time to work with. Brainstorm solutions to rid yourself of it. If driving in traffic is a huge stressor, perhaps shifting your driving time or listening to engaging audiobooks can help. If you don't get along with your boss, you may not be able to do much about that stress, but you can reshape how you handle it.

STAND STRONG ADRENAL SUPPORT TINCTURE

This is a strong adrenal tonic to rebuild balance in those who often feel stressed or "adrenalized." Adrenalized is that feeling when something small happens, but it triggers a huge physical response such as shaking, heart racing, stomach clenching, or the like. Remove the licorice root from this formula if you are experiencing hypertension.

2 tablespoons (30 ml) rhodiola bark tincture	YIELD: 4 ounces (120 ml)
4 teaspoons (20 ml) schizandra berry tincture	Combine all ingredients in a 4-ounce
4 teaspoons (20 ml) ashwagandha root tincture	(120 ml) amber dropper bottle.
4 teaspoons (20 ml) burdock root tincture	Take 1 dropperful 3 times per day for
4 teaspoons (20 ml) eleuthero root tincture	6 to 12 weeks.
2 teaspoons (10 ml) licorice root tincture	

PEACE AND CALM TEA

Nourishing the central nervous system will calm your mind and your perspective on the day's events. Drink as often as you'd like if you'd like a peaceful day.

1 ounce (28 g) dried passionflower leaf	YIELD: 4 ounces (112 g)
1 ounce (28 g) dried skullcap leaf	Combine all ingredients; store in a glass
1 ounce (28 g) dried chamomile flowers	jar. Steep 1 teaspoon (1.5 g) per cup of hot
½ ounce (14 g) dried catnip leaf	water for 8 to 10 minutes as needed.
¼ ounce (7 g) dried lavender flowers	
¼ ounce (7 g) dried rose petals	

RELAX NOW TINCTURE

For when you are "in it" and can recognize your need to take a step back and breathe.

2 tablespoons (30 ml) passionflower leaf tincture	**YIELD:** 4 ounces (120 ml)
2 tablespoons (30 ml) celery seed tincture	Combine all ingredients in a 4-ounce
4 teaspoons (20 ml) kava rhizome tincture	(120 ml) amber dropper bottle.
4 teaspoons (20 ml) California poppy flowers tincture	Take 2 dropperfuls as needed.
2 teaspoons (10 ml) nettle leaf tincture	
2 teaspoons (10 ml) hop flowers tincture	

TUMMY TENSION SALVE

Some of us hold all our stress and tension in our stomach. Using this salve topically will help alleviate the tightness held in the abdomen due to stress.

16 ounces (475 ml) olive oil	**YIELD:** 16 ounces (475 ml)
½ ounce (14 g) dried agrimony leaf	Place oil and herbs in a slow cooker; turn
½ ounce (14 g) dried skullcap leaf	heat to low and steep for 1 day. Strain and
¼ ounce (7 g) dried hop flowers	add beeswax. Stir until beeswax is melted,
1 to 2 ounces (28 to 56 g) grated beeswax	applying gentle heat if needed. Pour
	mixture into storage containers and let
	completely cool. Seal, label, and store in a
	cool, dark place. Apply as needed to abdomen to relieve stress held in the stomach
	or apply twice daily, morning and night.

ANXIETY RELEASE TINCTURE

Fear associated with nervousness is different from stress. It can lead to a sense of panic. This formula is focused on calming both the physical and mental aspects of anxiety.

2 tablespoons (30 ml) skullcap leaf tincture	**YIELD:** 4 ounces (120 ml)
4 teaspoons (20 ml) oat straw tincture	Combine all ingredients in a 4-ounce
4 teaspoons (20 ml) California poppy tincture	(120 ml) amber dropper bottle. Take
2 teaspoons (10 ml) agrimony leaf tincture	2 dropperfuls as needed.
4 teaspoons (20 ml) catnip leaf tincture	
4 teaspoons (20 ml) celery seed tincture	

MONKEY MIND TEA

The monkey mind typically arises for me right as I lay down to sleep. Sometimes it's first thing in the morning. Either of these times, I'd much rather be in a relaxed state instead of having my mind feeling as though it's in the starting blocks of a race. This tea helps hush that monkey and get it back into its cage.

1 ounce (28 g) dried skullcap leaf ½ ounce (14 g) dried oat straw ½ ounce (14 g) dried lemon balm leaf 1 ounce (28 g) dried ginger root	YIELD: 3 ounces (84 g) Combine all ingredients; store in a glass jar. To make a cup of tea, steep 1 to 2 teaspoons (1.5 to 3 g) per 1 cup (235 ml) of hot water for 8 to 10 minutes, as needed.

MORNING GIDDY UP CUP

Here's a new alternative to the morning routine with natural pick-me-ups.

1 ounce (28 g) dried ginkgo leaf 1 ounce (28 g) dried chicory root roasted ½ ounce (14 g) dried licorice root ½ ounce (14 g) dried gotu kola leaf ½ ounce (14 g) dried maca root	YIELD: 4 ounces (112 g) Combine all ingredients; store in a glass jar. Use 1 to 3 teaspoons (1.5 to 4.5 g) mixture per 1 cup (235 ml) of hot water. Let steep for 10 minutes; strain and drink.

CALM QUICK SHOT

This is an instant relaxer for when you are at home and ready to chill out.

3 tablespoons (45 ml) kava tincture 3 tablespoons (45 ml) oat straw tincture 3 tablespoons (45 ml) skullcap tincture	YIELD: 4 ounces (120 ml) Combine ingredients in a 4-ounce (120 ml) bottle. Take as ½-ounce (14 ml) shot as needed.

BEDTIME SHUT DOWN TINCTURE

Say goodnight, as this blend is sure to help you fall asleep quicker than normal.

2 tablespoons (30 ml) hop flowers tincture 2 tablespoons (30 ml) hawthorn berries tincture 2 tablespoons (30 ml) skullcap tincture 2 tablespoons (30 ml) chamomile tincture	YIELD: 4 ounces (120 ml) Combine all ingredients in a 4-ounce (120 ml) amber dropper bottle. Take 1 to 2 dropperfuls 30 minutes before bed and 1 dropperful as you slip between the covers.

BLADDER FREQUENCY, CYSTITIS, AND INTERSTITIAL CYSTITIS

Bladder issues can arise at almost any age and can be caused by a multitude of variances. Most arise from bladder irritation caused by diet, sex, muscle weakness, pregnancy, systemic pathologies (diabetes), medications, or hygiene failure. Some are triggered purely by emotional upset. I remember one young woman who complained of bladder frequency, irritation, and urgency with no infection. I asked her what she did for a living. She replied that she was a barista. I asked if she drank coffee. All day, was her reply. I recommended sticking to one cup and replacing coffee with water for the rest of the day. Within days, she was symptom free. Never underestimate the importance of examining your life and lifestyle choices when faced with new concerns.

TONE UP BLADDER SUPPORT TINCTURE

There are many times throughout our lives when our bladder isn't as strong as we'd like it to be. Diet is important, but blame ligament laxity most of the time. This formula works to strengthen and tone the system.

2 tablespoons (30 ml) buchu tincture	**YIELD:** 4 ounces (120 ml)
2 tablespoons (30 ml) nettle leaf tincture	Combine all ingredients in a 4-ounce
2 tablespoons (30 ml) red raspberry leaf tincture	(120 ml) amber dropper bottle. Take 1
2 tablespoons (30 ml) fenugreek tincture	dropperful 3 times per day for 6 to 8 weeks.

INTERSTITIAL CYSTITIS SUPPORT TINCTURE

This tincture is recommended for bladder frequency, pain, and urgency with no infection present.

2 tablespoons (30 ml) buchu tincture	**YIELD:** 4 ounces (120 ml)
2 tablespoons (30 ml) burdock seed tincture	Combine all ingredients in a 4-ounce
4 teaspoons (20 ml) lady's mantle tincture	(120 ml) amber dropper bottle.
4 teaspoons (20 ml) goldenrod tincture	Take 1 dropperful 3 times per day for
2 teaspoons (10 ml) catnip tincture	8 to 12 weeks.
2 teaspoons (10 ml) pipsissewa tincture	

CYSTITIS PREVENTATIVE TEA

Some women are more prone to bladder infections than others. This formula was created just for them, to keep the tract clean and encourage proper pH balance.

1 ounce (28 g) dried corn silk	YIELD: 6 ounces (168 g)
1 ounce (28 g) dried dandelion leaf	Make medicinal strength tea (see page
½ ounce (14 g) dried nettle leaf	245); drink 3 cups per day for 8 weeks.
½ ounce (14 g) dried goldenrod leaf	
½ ounce (14 g) dried cleavers leaf	
2 ounces (56 g) dried peppermint leaf	

BLADDER SOOTHE TEA

Drink this formula at the first sign of bladder irritation to soothe the membranes.

2 ounces (56 g) dried marshmallow root	YIELD: 6 ounces (168 g)
1 ounce (28 g) dried cleavers	Combine all ingredients; store in a glass jar.
1 ounce (28 g) dried chickweed	For a cup of tea, steep 2 teaspoons (3 g) per
1 ounce (28 g) dried chamomile	1 cup (235 ml) of hot water for 10 minutes.
½ ounce (14 g) dried lavender	

ANTIBACTERIAL BLADDER SUPPORT TINCTURE

This is formulated for urinary tract infections but must be used with regular consistency to be effective. Try this formula at the first sign of possible infection in an attempt to nip it in the bud. If no improvement occurs or your symptoms worsen within 24 hours, seek professional care. Urinary tract infections need to be diagnosed and treated professionally. An untreated or worsening infection can be life-threatening.

1½ tablespoons (25 ml) goldenseal tincture	YIELD: 4 ounces (120 ml)
4 teaspoons (20 ml) echinacea root tincture	Combine all ingredients in a 4-ounce
4 teaspoons (20 ml) uva ursi tincture	(120 ml) amber dropper bottle. Take 2
4 teaspoons (20 ml) dandelion leaf tincture	dropperfuls every 3 hours for 3 to 5 days.
1 tablespoon (15 ml) pipsissewa tincture	
2 teaspoons (10 ml) Oregon grape root tincture	
2 teaspoons (10 ml) cleavers tincture	

THYROID HEALTH

Thyroid health and the pathologies of it in the twenty-first century are extremely common and well known. Why are so many people affected worldwide? There are many theories, including the rise in autoimmunity. Autoimmunity occurs when healthy systems go awry. Healthy tissues are attacked by their own kind, which leads to a degradation in function. Some research points to genetics and environmental factors as the causes; others indicate processed and genetically modified food consumption. In my clinical experience, I've seen direct correlation between digestion health and thyroid function. Discuss the recipes below with your health care practitioner before administration if you are currently taking thyroid medications. Taking herbs that support the thyroid in conjunction with thyroid medication needs to be supervised so as to not overstimulate or depress thyroid function.

THYROID SUPPORT CAPSULES

This blend is for the normally operating thyroid; it provides key ingredients to optimize the gland's health and function.

1 ounce (28 g) kelp powder	YIELD: 200 capsules
½ ounce (14 g) fennel seed powder	Combine all powders in a bowl. Use the
½ ounce (14 g) parsley leaf powder	mixture to fill empty vegetable capsules.
½ ounce (14 g) barberry powder	Take 2 capsules once daily upon rising.
½ ounce (14 g) cleavers powder	

CALMING OVERACTIVITY TINCTURE

This tincture is used as a tonic to reduce a hyperactive thyroid and support overall function. Discuss with you practitioner before initiating.

1 tablespoon (15 ml) motherwort leaf tincture	YIELD: 2 ounces (60 ml)
1 tablespoon (15 ml) goldenseal root tincture	Combine all ingredients in a 2-ounce
2 teaspoons (10 ml) bugleweed herb tincture	(60 ml) amber dropper bottle. Take 10
2 teaspoons (10 ml) black walnut hulls tincture	drops 3 times per day for 8 to 12 weeks.
2 teaspoons (10 ml) lemon balm leaf tincture	

THYROID SUPPORT OIL

This oil is recommended for any dysfunction of the thyroid gland (or any gland for that matter) to relieve congestion and stagnation.

1 ounce (28 g) dried mullein leaf

⅓ ounce (9 g) dried lobelia leaf

1 to 2 cups (235 to 475 ml) olive oil

Sweet orange essential oil

YIELD: 1½ cups (355 ml)

Preheat oven to 170°F (77°C). Place herbs in a glass baking dish and pour olive oil over them, making sure to leave 1 to 2 inches (3 to 5 cm) at the top. Bake for 4 hours, stirring occasionally. Allow to cool, and then strain into a storage container. Add sweet orange essential oil and mix well. Apply to neck at thyroid area each night before bed.

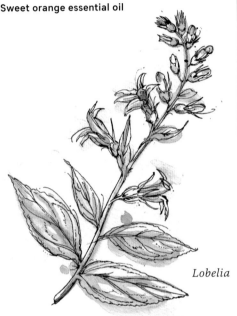

Lobelia

THYROID FATIGUE TINCTURE

My patients often share with me the extreme fatigue they experience on a daily basis. I visualize it as walking through knee-high mud all day. This formula was blended for them. Although it doesn't specifically treat the thyroid, it supports the thyroid-adrenal axis to give them a bit of a boost while working to heal the underlying problem.

2 teaspoons (10 ml) spirulina tincture

1 teaspoon (5 ml) eleuthero root tincture

1 teaspoon (5 ml) alfalfa leaf tincture

1 teaspoon (5 ml) nettle leaf tincture

1 teaspoon (5 ml) licorice root tincture

YIELD: 1 ounce (28 ml)

Combine all ingredients in a 1-ounce (28 ml) amber dropper bottle. Take 1 to 2 dropperfuls when you need a pick-me-up.

CARDIAC HEALTH

As women, we often lead with our hearts—literally and figuratively. The need to care for our cardiac system is more evident than ever as heart disease rises. It is the number one-cause of death for women in America. Naturally, I believe our mental and spiritual health is equally as important as our physical health, and there should be practices in place to support both. Sometimes I lie down to bed and realize I haven't taken a deep breath all day. Although the heart naturally pumps oxygen throughout our body, if we are holding our breath, that transport is greatly diminished. Start and end your day with ten full, deep breathes. Do them as you are waiting at stoplights or taking other pauses during your day. Whenever you can, remember this vital relationship between the lungs and heart. Place your hand over your heart to initiate a reconnection. In many acupuncture sessions, when I've needled a point over the heart, it has elicited great emotional release.

In Chinese medicine philosophy, the pericardium, the sheath that covers the heart, is considered the heart protector. It protects the heart by determining what will and will not be allowed in. As you can imagine, there is plenty that doesn't make its way across the threshold and is held by the pericardium. We need to find ways to release this emotional and physical buildup. We can hold an enormous amount and often don't ever release it.

HEART HEALTH TONIC TEA

This tea is a wonderful way to bring healing intention to the Empress of our body.

1 ounce (28 g) dried motherwort

1 ounce (28 g) dried hawthorn berry

½ ounce (14 g) dried hawthorn leaf and flower

½ ounce (14 g) dried ginger

1 ounce (28 g) dried hibiscus

½ ounce (14 g) dried rosehips

½ ounce (14 g) dried raspberry pieces

YIELD: 5 ounces (140 g)

Combine all ingredients; store in a glass jar. Make medicinal strength (see page 245) each evening; drink 3 cups per day for 8 to 12 weeks.

CIRCULATION SUPPORT TINCTURE

Supporting the circulation system means the heart doesn't have to work quite as hard. By nourishing its vessels, you are nourishing your entire cardiac system.

2 teaspoons (10 ml) safflower tincture

2 teaspoons (10 ml) hawthorn berry tincture

1 teaspoon (5 ml) ginkgo leaf tincture

1 teaspoon (5 ml) maca tincture

1 dropperful cayenne tincture

YIELD: 1 ounce (28 ml)

Combine all ingredients in a 1-ounce (28 ml) amber dropper bottle. Take 1 dropperful twice daily.

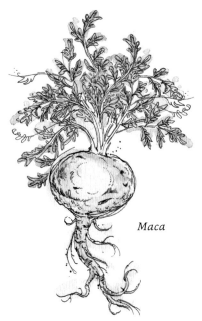

Maca

HYPERHEART TINCTURE

Sometimes food, stress, or digestive upset can lead to heart palpitations, or a fluttering feeling in the heart. If you've been examined by your physician and all is well, yet you continue to experience these symptoms, this formula is worth a try.

2 teaspoons (10 ml) skullcap leaf tincture

2 teaspoons (10 ml) chamomile flower tincture

1 teaspoon (5 ml) catnip leaf tincture

1 teaspoon (5 ml) wild cherry bark tincture

YIELD: 1 ounce (28 ml)

Combine all ingredients in a 1-ounce (28 ml) amber dropper bottle. Take 1 to 2 dropperfuls as needed when you feel your heart picking up the pace.

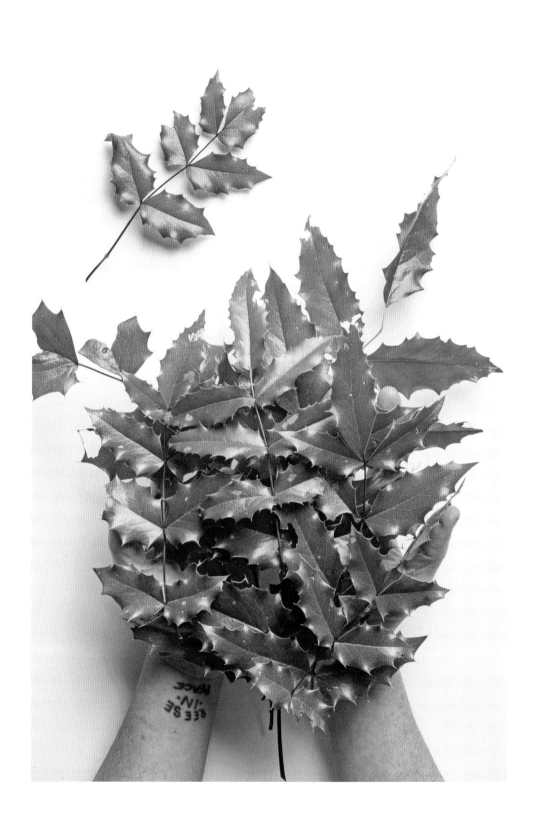

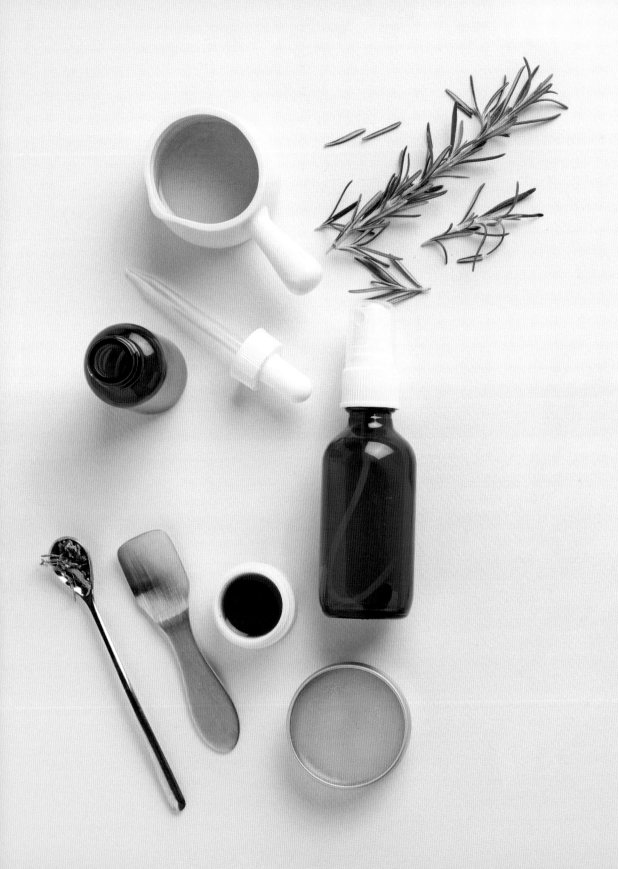

CHAPTER 8

Making
Herbal Medicine

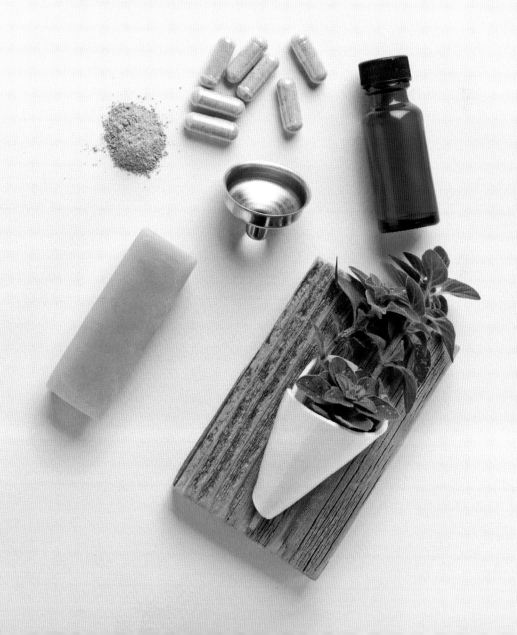

I T'S ONE THING TO LEARN ABOUT HERBAL MEDICINE and another to feel confident enough to *make* herbal medicine. Because you are just beginning, I suggest always starting small. Anything can be made in smaller proportions; simply reduce the ingredients by half or even a quarter. The learning curve on tea blending is probably the steepest. Just like cooking, you are dealing with a plethora of flavors and potential palates, and learning how to navigate them takes time. But the rest of the herbal medicine applications can be made with surprising ease.

Always keep a medicine-making journal or logbook. Record herb amounts used, all ingredients, and their proportions. Be sure to include dates as well. If you are making a tincture or herbal oil, you'll want to know when it was made and when to strain it. Having an idea of how old something is can be helpful as well. If something doesn't turn out right, be sure to make notes so you can troubleshoot the next time.

Storage Tips

Glass makes for great storage vessels, so start saving those jelly and spaghetti jars now. I prefer to store all my herbs and herbal products in a cool, dry place, away from direct sunlight.

TINCTURES

Tincture making has been recorded for almost five thousand years. Alcohol was most likely first introduced in China with the fermentation of rice, honey, and fruit; and the ancient Egyptians had concrete knowledge of how to preserve food, including plants. There is also evidence that cordials were present at that time; they can be considered the first record of "tinctures." Cordials are made from herbs, and often fruit, left to soak in alcohol and strained at a later date. By modern definition, a cordial is an alcoholic drink that contains a minimum of 2.5 percent sugar by weight. Typically, this sugar is derived from a combination of fermentation and fruit.

In short, a tincture is a plant medicine for which the plant material is saturated in alcohol long enough to allow the cellular structures to break down and the alcohol to extract the medicinal constituents. You can use vodka, wine, brandy, and 99 proof varieties. Because knowledge of specific solvent ranges is necessary if you are using something besides vodka, vodka is used most often. If alcohol is not an option, I would suggest using teas or capsules for oral dosing. There is a small pool of herbs that can be extracted in vegetable glycerin or apple cider vinegar, but their drawing power is minimal compared to alcohol.

BASIC TINCTURE

2 tablespoons (9 g) fresh herbs or 2 teaspoons (3 g) dried herbs	YIELD: 1 ounce (28 ml)
1 ounce (28 ml) vodka	Place herbs in a 1-ounce (28 ml) jar with firm-fitting lid; add vodka. Close the lid tightly and shake for 20 seconds. Store in a cool, dark place for 14 to 21 days, shaking each day. Strain and store in a 1-ounce (28 ml) amber dropper bottle in a cool, dry area, preferably away from direct sunlight.
	Note: When blending tinctures, use a graduated cylinder to measure out the designated amount. Pour it directly into the blend's dropper bottle. (Tinctures are dispensed by dropperfuls, so they are always best stored in an amber dropper bottle.) Close and gently shake. Most tinctures have a shelf life of up to ten years.

HERBAL CAPSULES

Herbal capsules are extremely convenient and easy to make. Making them yourself also gives you control over what goes into them. I love using herbs individually at times, as I think the body responds wonderfully when working one-on-one with plants. Making your own capsules allows for this creative choice to use the medicine how you wish. I also love making my own capsules, because then I don't have to pay for all the excessive packaging that often drives up the cost of purchased products. I recommend using kosher-grade vegetable cellulose capsules when making your own herbal medicine. They are more readily broken down in the body and easier to digest overall. Not to mention you remove the animal aspect; standard gelatin capsules are a by-product of the meat and leather industries.

The capsule recipes in this book call for powdered herbs. This makes it much easier to blend herbs together and put into the empty vegetable capsules. You can purchase them in powdered form, or you can grind down dried herbs yourself if you have something like a Vitamix to get somewhat of a fine powder. Most capsule recipes make approximately 100 to 200 capsules. Roughly 1 ounce (28 g) of powdered herb makes 100 capsules. Capsules come in various sizes, with the most common being a size 0 or a 00.

There are two ways to make capsules. You can purchase a capsule machine, like Cap-M-Quik, or produce them home-style. Capsule machines cost about twenty dollars and typically make 100 capsules at a time; they really are worth the investment. Read the manufacturer's instructions for specifics, but in general you insert the capsule bottoms into the filling tray and pour the herbal powder onto the tray. Then you use the provided powder spreader and move the powder around until the capsules are full. You then lower the top tray and put the tops on. It's easy. Just as easy, although a bit more time-consuming, is making capsules home-style. Put your capsules in one bowl and your herbal powder in another. Then, open a capsule and simply scoop the top and the bottom toward each other in the powder to fill it. Cap it together and continue. Your hands will get dirty, and you need be sure to keep all moisture away from the process. After a bit of practice, you'll get proficient and fast.

HERBAL OILS

There is nothing prettier then herbal oils sitting in the sunshine. Their colors become dramatic over time as the plant material diffuses its medicine into the carrier oil. St. John's wort is a great plant to work with the first time you make fresh herbal oil; the red color it turns is extremely rewarding. I also enjoy working with fresh poplar buds toward the end of winter—they mark the hopeful return of spring, and their fragrance is intoxicating. Remember that herbal oils are not the same as essential oils. Essential oils are procured through a distillation process; herbal oils are made through a maceration process with the addition of heat.

There are two approaches to making herbal oils. One is through solar infusion, which utilizes the heat from the sun during a maceration period. The other utilizes artificial heat to draw out the medicinal constituents. Artificial heat sources include the oven, a slow cooker, or a double boiler. Typically, fresh material is processed using the solar method and dried material using artificial heat.

SOLAR INFUSION METHOD

½ cup (36 g) fresh
herb material

4 ounces (120 ml)
olive oil

YIELD: 4 ounces (120 ml)

Place herbs and olive oil in a 4-ounce (120 ml) mason jar; tighten
the lid. Give the jar a good shake and set in the sun, ensuring
a consistent temperature above 75°F (24°C). (**Note:** Check the
weather! If you don't live where there will be consistent work
temperatures overnight, use the oven method instead.) Let it sit
for 2 to 3 weeks, shaking daily. If you notice precipitates at the
bottom of the jar, this is water being pulled from the plant material.
Open the jar and use a baster to suck the material out of the jar.
Alternatively, suck out the precipitates and then put the entire
contents of the jar into a saucepan. Bring to an almost boil before
turning off the stove and returning the mixture to the jar
to complete the solar infusion process.

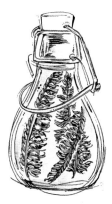

ARTIFICIAL HEATING METHOD

¼ cup (18 g) dried
herb material (Try
calendula to start;
it makes a great
base herb oil.)

4 ounces (120 ml)
olive oil

YIELD: 4 ounces (120 ml)

Place all ingredients in a small glass baking pan. Set oven to 170°F
(77°C) degrees or the lowest setting on your oven. (**Note:** If
your oven's lowest temperature setting is 200°F (93°C) degrees,
bake the herbs with the oven door slightly ajar.) Bake for 4 hours,
stirring occasionally. Allow to cool and then strain into a 4-ounce
(120 ml) amber bottle. Store in a cool, dark place for future use.
To ensure longer shelf life, you can add essential oils as a preservative; 10 to 20 drops is plenty for a 4-ounce (120 ml) bottle.

SALVES

Salves are an extremely handy medicine to have around the house. I'm not sure at what point we as a society became so bad at self-care, but I believe that salves can be a starting point to return to that practice. Burn yourself while cooking? Dab some salve on it. Is a hangnail on your thumb causing it to throb? Dab some salve on it. Is a crack in your heel making it hard to walk? Dab some salve on it. The simple practice of acknowledging that something needs care can shift us—and perhaps grow into shifting our communities—to a more generalized state of self-care.

You can use a salve for almost anything. Generally, salves are used for cuts, burns, wounds, bites, stings, and the like; but get creative. Anything that can be used in herbal medicine can be turned into a salve. One of my favorites is a moon salve that I made for menstrual cramping. Taking a moment to rub a bit of salve onto the abdomen over a cramping uterus allows us to relax into the pain. I know that sounds off—you may have no interest in relaxing into the pain of your menstrual cramping. What I'm trying to say is that if you take a moment to acknowledge pain, it has the opportunity to shift. It is when we ignore pain, work through it, and act as though it isn't happening that it often gets worse.

Although essential oils can be used to extend salves' shelf lives, most oils and salves without essential oils will go rancid after six months.

BASIC SALVE

3½ ounces (104 ml) herbal oil of your choice. What you decide is based on what the salve's purpose will be. If you want a general all-purpose salve for cuts and burn, use calendula or lavender flower.

½ ounce (14 g) beeswax

YIELD: 4 ounces (120 ml)

Gently warm the herbal oil over low heat; stir in beeswax until melted. It's best to stir continuously as the beeswax melts. Pour salve into a 4-ounce (120 ml) jar; allow it to cool completely before closing.

After pouring the salve into the jar, you may wish to add essential oils to extend your salve's shelf life. For a 4-ounce (120 ml) jar, add 20 to 40 drops; lavender essential oil is a good choice for an all-purpose first-aid salve—it is antimicrobial, antibacterial, and healing for burns.

SYRUPS

A syrup is truly my favorite way to take herbal medicine. Although not all herbs translate into a syrup, many do. Herbs whose medicines are derived from alkaloids will need the alcohol in the tincture method to draw out their healing qualities, but herbs with water-soluble healing properties can be made into syrups.

Syrups are also a great way to introduce kids to herbs. Because syrups are either honey or sugar based, their sweetness is a natural attractant. Kids also seems to be naturally drawn to the flavor of herbs, particularly the sweet nature of healing berries and roots. Every fall, we collect fresh elderberries as a family and make a yearly batch of elderberry syrup. Including your children in this ritual connects them to the medicine they take.

Syrups, like salves, can be an herbal application for almost anything. Some examples of different syrups you can make include iron building, mineralizing, female balancing, liver supporting, immune support, and stress reducing.

BASIC SYRUP

½ cup (36 g) fresh or ¼ cup (18 g) dried herbal material

4 ounces (120 ml) honey or 2 to 4 ounces (56 to 112 g) cane sugar

Apple cider vinegar (optional)

YIELD: 8 ounces (235 ml)

Add the herbs to 8 to 10 ounces (235 to 285 ml) of water in a saucepan. Cover the pan and simmer on low, with lid slightly ajar, until the water is reduced approximately by half. Strain well. Put the strained liquid back into the now-clean saucepan. Add honey or cane sugar. Place over low heat and stir until the honey or sugar is completely dissolved. I often continue stirring and gently warming for 5 additional minutes after the last remnants are dissolved. At this point, I typically add a splash of apple cider vinegar for further shelf life stability and flavor. This is not a requirement, as sugar/honey is a natural preservative. Store syrup in an 8-ounce (235 ml) bottle for future use. It can be kept in the refrigerator for 3 to 6 months or 2 to 3 months unrefrigerated.

POULTICES

A poultice is as natural an herbal remedy as you are ever going to find. It is a front-line application, with the placement of fresh or dried plant material directly onto the skin. A great example is the use of fresh comfrey leaves on a broken arm. Simply collect the fresh leaves and put them in a large bowl; add a splash of hot water. Use a pestle to gentle crush the leaves, but leave them whole. Wrap the arm over and over with the leaves. Leave the poultice on overnight if possible. Even if you have a cast, you can use this poultice above or below the cast to aid in the healing process; just make sure you don't get water or plant material under the cast itself. Stuffing muslin or cotton into the cast gaps can prevent this.

I also use poultices for bed sores. Bed sores occur when someone is bed bound and the weight of his or her body causes lack of circulation in the area where the body is lying on the mattress. Bed sores can be excruciating and, left untreated, can quickly become infected. I mash up herbs such as goldenseal, calendula, chickweed, and myrrh with my mortar and pestle; add a touch of hot water, allow the poultice to cool slightly, and then pack the bed sore with it. This helps fight infection, promotes closure of the sore, and helps cool down inflammation.

YELLOW JACKET STING POULTICE

The following ingredients are readily available during late summer, when yellow jackets are in a frenzy preparing for winter and when the human world and their world often collide.

2 fresh plantain leaves 1 fresh chickweed stem	YIELD: 1 poultice Put all 3 leaves in a bowl; add a touch of hot water. Mix and mash until leaves are really broken up. Add enough water so the leaves stick together and an herb cake can be formed. Apply this directly onto the sting site, doing your best to ensure the stinger is out. Not to worry if you are not sure, as the poultice will draw out the stinger if it is still present. Wrap the poultice with muslin or medical gauze to secure it in place. Refresh every 3 to 4 hours, but you should begin to feel relief immediately.

FOMENTATION

A fomentation is another topical application. It's better used when the area you are treating is large or uneven, making the use of a poultice cumbersome. A fomentation is the steep infusion of herbs. I use 4 tablespoons (18 g) herbs to 16 ounces (475 ml) of water. Make it similarly to a tea, in that if your ingredients are leaves, an infusion is fine, but I tend to allow a fomentation to steep for 1 to 2 hours if time allows. If you are using roots, simmer for 10 to 12 minutes; then turn off the heat and allow the mixture to infuse for 1 hour, covered. After straining, soak a cotton cloth in the fomentation, wring it mostly out, and apply to the afflicted area. This is a great treatment for abdomen or cramping pain, as the combination of the warmth and the herbs often brings quick comfort to pain. I also use fomentations with my kids when they have colds, placing it on their chest or upper back. Sleep tends to result quickly.

SPRAINED ANKLE FOMENTATION

4 tablespoons (18 g) witch hazel leaf	YIELD: 1 treatment
	Steep the witch hazel in 16 ounces (475 ml) of hot water, covered, for 1 to 2 hours.
	Strain the leaves from the infusion and warm it over low heat. Soak a cotton cloth in the infusion and wrap the ankle. Elevate the ankle and rest.

SITZ BATHS AND TOPICAL WASHES

These are topical applications used to treat specific areas of the body. Sitz baths focus on the pelvic regions, including the vaginal and anal areas. They are great for healing vaginal tissues, treating hemorrhoids, and moving circulation in the pelvic bowl. Topical washes are much like fomentations, but instead of soaking a cloth in the infusion and applying it to the body, you soak the body part in the infusion itself. Obviously, not every body part can easily be soaked, hence the need for fomentations. But body parts such as the hands or feet can greatly benefit from direct submersion in an herbal infusion. Both applications allow for direct and consistent immersion. They are made as you would make a fomentation, using more herbs per water ratio— 4 tablespoons (18 g) per 16 ounces (475 ml) water—and allowing for a longer infusion, 1 to 2 hours or longer. Because these applications are rarely needed in an acute situation, you can allow them to infuse for a longer time, ideally 4 to 6 hours. If you have that much time, you can actually infuse your roots instead of simmering them, as the longer infusion time will allow for breakdown of roots and bark. This is helpful when you are using a combination of herbs that include leaves, flowers, roots, and bark.

I recommend warming the infusion before soaking, but sometimes a cool application is best, such as with hot skin conditions. Put the infusion into the appropriate basin and soak.

TEA

What a great place to end this section. In fact, why not stop for a moment and go make a nice cup of tea before you read on! What is it about tea that naturally promotes relaxation? Perhaps it is the ritual, the scent of the steam as it rolls off the cup. It's true; I'm obsessed with tea and addicted to the practice of it. My hope is that you soon will be too!

There are two reasons we drink tea. One is for pleasure; the other is for medicine. The blending of beverage teas takes practice, but there is no reason not to dive in. Learn which herbs you really like and begin blending two or three at a time. Learn their individual flavors and what happens when you blend them with other herbs. Learn what happens when you steep certain herbs too long or when you put in more of one herb versus another. This is the art and science of combining herbs and flavors. Take diligent notes and continue to perfect your home blends. Soon enough, your friends will be asking for your recipes!

The other reason we drink herbal teas is to heal or bring balance back into the body. Most of us are familiar with Traditional Medicinals tea, originally created by herbalist and one of my mentors, Rosemary Gladstar. Found in most grocery stores, Traditional Medicinals was one of the first companies to bring the idea of healing tea to the general public. Throat Coat and Smooth Move are almost household names today because of Rosemary's work.

When first beginning to use herbs for medicinal use, it is best to familiarize yourself with one herb at a time. Try a nervine such as passionflower or skullcap to discover its flavor and its actions on your body. Then try adding one additional herb. In this case, try blending passionflower with chamomile and again investigate the same questions. You can read books about herbs all day long, but until you begin working and using them, you know very little.

Most of the teas in this book are formulated to make 4 ounces (120 ml) of tea. Drink 2 to 3 cups a day of medicinal tea when trying to create a physiological change in the body. This is typically continued for 6 to 12 weeks. Usually 2 to 4 pounds (1 to 2 kg) of tea will provide you with a 30-day supply of 3 daily cups of medicinal-strength tea. Four ounces of tea will make roughly 80 cups if you're using only 1 to 2 teaspoons (1.5 to 3 g) per cup. To blend them, place all ingredients in a nice large mixing bowl. Use a big wooden spoon to gently blend all the herbs together until evenly mixed. Kept in an air-tight glass jar, away from heat and direct sunlight, teas can last up to a year.

You will want to make the medicinal herb teas in this book at medicinal strength unless otherwise indicated.

MEDICINAL STRENGTH TEA

4 to 5 tablespoons (18 to 22.5 g) herbs	YIELD: 1 treatment
	Put the herbs in a 1-quart (1 L) jar or a saucepan and pour hot water over them. Boiling water is fine, but the ideal temperature is 190°F (88°C). Close the jar, or place a lid on the pan, and allow to steep overnight. In the morning, strain the herbs. This is your daily allotment of herbal tea to reach a desired medicinal dosage. You can divide this into 3 cups per day, or sip on it throughout the day. You can drink it hot or cold, unless you are focusing on warming a system or body part, in which case it is best hot. I also think tea drunk after meals or before bed is best hot.

A general guide to steeping:

- For teas with leaves and flowers—steep for 8 to 12 minutes, covered.
- For teas with roots and barks—simmer for 10 to 12 minutes, covered.
- For teas with leaves or flowers combined with roots or bark—simmer for 10 to 12 minutes; turn off the heat. Add an additional 1 to 2 teaspoon (1.5 to 3 g) of the herbal mixture, cover, and allow to steep an additional 10 minutes.

RESOURCES
General Dosing Guidelines for Herbal Medicine

These are by no means hard-and-fast rules, but they are offered here as a simple guideline for dosing applications.

Please keep in mind that herbs are best used in frequent smaller doses throughout the day rather than occasional large doses.

Medicinal Teas

3 cups per day, or 1 quart (1 L) spread out throughout the day

Capsules

ACUTE: 2 to 3 capsules 3 to 4 times per day

CHRONIC/TONIC: 2 capsules 1 to 2 times per day

Tinctures

ACUTE: 2 dropperfuls every 2 to 3 hours for 1 to 2 days, then 2 dropperfuls 2 to 3 times per day for 5 days

CHRONIC/TONIC: 1 dropperful 3 times per day

Poultices/Fomentation

TYPICALLY USED FOR ACUTE CONDITIONS: Apply 2 times per day, 30 minutes with gentle heat

Children

TEAS AND SYRUPS: Teaspoon doses 3 to 6 times per day, depending on case

GLYCERIN TINCTURES: 1 dropperful 3 to 4 times per day

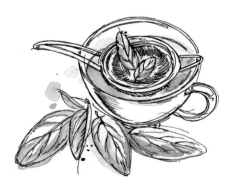

Where to Purchase Quality Herbs

Purchasing quality herbs will make or break your herbal experience. When I first moved to Portland, Oregon, there were no herb shops close by in the Portland metro area. There was one store that had herbs, but they were not organic; when I stood before the wall of herbs, they were all almost the same color. That isn't normal. Herbs should vibrate their energy through their colors, smells, and flavors. When you go to any herb shop, open the jars; look at the herbs and smell them. You'll quickly know the difference between quality herbs and mass-produced product. An herb is only as good as its source, so choose high-quality herbs when you intend to use them as medicine. If the herb is not grown or processed correctly, it may look normal, but it will not contain the constituents necessary for healing. The processing piece is extremely important, particularly when using dried herbs. Each herb needs to be processed and handled in particular ways or the medicinal constituents could be destroyed. I've seen this time and time again, especially from big companies with no other agenda than to make a profit from the herbal growth trend. They produce countless products that, when tested, have virtually nothing in them. If you really want to do your homework, ask companies for certificates of analysis for their herbs. These certificates demonstrate the medicinal quality of their herbs and their quality control. I recommend the following companies.

FOR SMALLER QUANTITY HERBAL PURCHASES

Fettle Botanic Supply & Counsel www.fettlebotanic.com

FOR LARGER QUANTITIES (1-POUND [455 g] INCREMENTS)

Mountain Rose Herbs www.mountainroseherbs.com

Pacific Botanicals www.pacificbotanicals.com

Oregon's Wild Harvest www.oregonswildharvest.com

Herbalist Conferences, Societies, and Schools

Belonging to herbal organizations and attending herbal conferences can be very rewarding. Surrounding yourself with others who are passionate about herbs can catapult your learning experience. Search out herbalists in your community for grassroots learning as well as an opportunity to learn the flora and fauna of your specific region. Remember, the day-to-day ailments of each region most often have the appropriate healing plants growing nearby.

Herbal Conferences

If you love traveling and submerging into learning for two to four days at a time, seek out some of the annual herbal conferences around the country. Here are a few of my favorites.

Southeast Wise Women's Herbal Conference www.sewisewomen.com

Medicines from the Earth Herb Symposium www.botanicalmedicine.org

New England Women's Herbal Conference www.facebook.com/womensherbalconference

Pacific Women's Herbal Conference www.pacificwomensherbalconference.com

Northern California Women's Herbal Symposium www.womensherbalsymposium.org

Southwest Conference on Botanical Medicine www.botanicalmedicine.org

Breitenbush Herbal Conference www.breitenbushherbalconference.com

The Dandelion Seed Conference http://dandelionseedconference.weebly.com

Herbal Societies

American Herbalists Guild www.americanherbalistsguild.com

American Botanical Counsel http://abc.herbalgram.org

United Plant Savers www.unitedplantsavers.org

American Herbal Pharmacopoeia www.herbal-ahp.org

Herb Research Foundation www.herbs.org

Herbal Studies and Schools

For a complete and comprehensive list, visit www.herbnet.com/university_p1.htm

Blue Otter School of Herbal Medicine www.blueotterschool.com
A comprehensive school in northern California led by Karyn Sanders and Sarah Holmes.

California School of Herbal Studies http://cshs.com
Founded by Rosemary Gladstar; one of the United States's first schools of herbal studies.

Southwest School of Botanical Medicine http://swsbm.com
Founded by herbalist Michael Moore; continues through a distance-learning program.

EarthSong Herbals http://earthsongherbals.com
If you want to learn how to work with clients as an herbalist or herbal consultant, this is a great learning experience. It's one of the few that offers clinic experience.

Midwest School of Herbal Studies www.midwestherbalstudies.com
This school offers two programs: A one-year Western-Herbalism Certificate Program and a two-year Master-Herbalist Diploma Program.

Center for Herbal Studies www.herbalstudies.net
David Winston's Center for Herbal Studies is highly recommended.

New Mexico School of Natural Therapeutics http://nmsnt.org
You will get much more than just herbs from this experience. It offers a multidimensional approach to healing through the education of several modalities.

ArborVitae School of Traditional Herbalism https://arborvitaeny.com
In New York City, this is a three-year comprehensive program to study herbal medicine.

Dr. Christopher's School of Natural Healing www.schoolofnaturalhealing.com
Dr. Christopher's work has aided in the education of herbalism for many decades. The school offers a distance-learning program.

Rosemary Gladstar's The Science & Art of Herbal Medicine
https://scienceandartofherbalism.com
A wonderful foundational certification program in herbal medicine. It is self-learning through ten courses that include homework and projects to be completed. Or you can visit Sage Mountain for a hands-on course.

IN CLOSING

It is with gratitude that I bring this book to its end. Thank you for taking the time to read, laugh, and consider all that I've brought to these pages. My intention is to first and foremost offer hope, support, and herbal wisdom to those who are interested and in need. Herbs have provided so much for me in my life, with the greatest gift being powerfully peaceful moments of belonging and clarity. Secondly, it is my desire that anyone who reads this, no matter what gender, recognizes the beauty and power you hold. It is your strength that creates the path upon which you walk and the world that you weave. Be strong, be bold, and always follow your heart. Lastly, please love the plants. Speak kindly to them, thank them, and do everything possible to ensure their safety.

Kind regards,
Dr. JJ

ACKNOWLEDGMENTS

This book would not have been possible without having the resources, references, support, and guidance of all of the herbalists before me. Susun Weed once said to me, "What do you have to say that hasn't already been written?" While Susun can be a harsh critic, I respect her dearly and I thought long and hard about this. What I discovered was that while there may be many herbal books out there, it was my voice that I truly wanted to share, along with my experiences of using herbs. So thank you to all of those who came before me, a countless number, but in particular, Linda Quintana, Susun Weed, Rosemary Gladstar, Scott Kloos, David Hoffmann, and Jill Stansbury. Those who, despite resistance, forged ahead so that we all could benefit.

With deep gratitude, I thank Shawn Linehan, who photographed this book to make it as beautiful as it is. Your artistic eye and talent are, as always, a pure joy to work with.

Thank you to my husband, Brian, and mom, Jo, for caring for the kids to give me the time to hole up in the Hillsboro Public Library to get some quiet space to put the words on the page. And, of course, everyone at The Quarto Group, but particularly Jill Alexander, Meredith Quinn, and Marissa Giambrone for their dedication and commitment to making this book the best it could be.

Lastly: Thank you to the plants. It is your beauty and inspiration that keeps me in awe each and every day.

ABOUT THE AUTHOR

Dr. JJ Pursell is a board certified naturopathic physician and licensed acupuncturist and has worked with medicinal herbs for more than twenty-five years. She has taught and trained with herbalists all over the world but prefers the practice of close-to-home

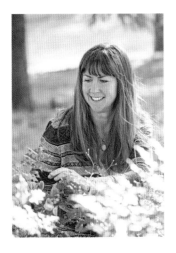

grown western herbs. Her Portland-based shop Fettle Botanic Supply & Counsel, once known as The Herb Shoppe, focuses on offering the most vital organic herbs available while sustaining local growers.

The author of *The Herbal Apothecary* and *The Herbal Book: 375 Herbal Recipes*, Dr. JJ is also a member of both the Oregon Association of Naturopathic Physicians and the American Association of Nurse Practitioners, contributing to events and policy opinion. She speaks across the country at expos, conventions, schools, and groups such as the New York Horticulture Society.

JJ and her shop have been featured in *Portland Monthly* magazine, *L Magazine* in New York City, several blogs and Tumblr sites, and on television and radio. She has her own YouTube channel for those who want to learn more about making herbal medicine.

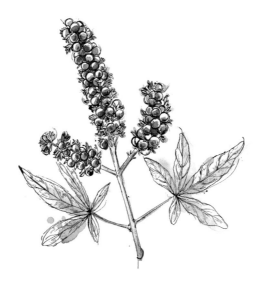

Index